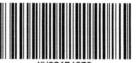

POETRY CHANGES LIVES

POETRY CHANGES LIVES

Daily Thoughts on History and Poetry

CHRISTOPHER BURN

POETRY CHANGES LIVES
First published in 2015
by DHH Publishing
The Old Joiners Shop
Skirling by Biggar, South Lanarkshire,
ML12 6HD
Scotland, UK

All rights reserved
© Christopher Burn, 2015
Christopher Burn is hereby identified as author
of this work in accordance with Section 77 of the Copyright,
Designs and Patents Act 1988

Cover design by Helen Wyllie
Cover photograph of Louis Blériot from the
George Grantham Bain Collection, US Library of Congress

A CIP record for this book is available from the British Library
ISBN   978-0-9934663-1-1

Foreword

Several months ago Chris asked me to edit this book. Not being an expert on what I thought of as daily instruction books, I hesitated. But then my curiosity and altruism got the better of me.

It has been a wonderful journey, reading about people and incidents both famous and infamous. Because of the nature of the book, one person or 'happening' a day or per page (like Martin Luther King, or the first flight across the Atlantic), you may well think it to be superficial, but the author almost always leads us to explore further.

He may recount a quirky or dramatic incident in one of his page-a-day accounts and all too often I would find myself looking up the day's subject in Wikipedia, checking the facts, being drawn into the history and of course learning more.

Following this intriguing historical offering we are then given a poem for each day. Some of them I love, some I struggle with and some, just a few, I don't much like. But I love the daily entertainment! Every page is thought provoking and the line at the foot of the page invites us to reflect on our own lives and how we would really like to be.

So all in all, each day offers us a gigantic package of fact, creativity and healthy introspection. It affects me, it makes me think, and I hope it will do the same for you.

Stephanie Wolfe Murray

For Margie, Alex, Johnnie and Annabel
Jo, Cathy and Rob
Alfie, Ben, Olivia, Oscar and Sophie.

Acknowledgments

Unprovided with original learning, unformed in the habits of thinking, unskilled in the arts of composition, I resolved to write a book.

Edward Gibbon

Gibbon is one of my heroes. He was not afraid to try doing things he knew little about. I wonder what he would have made of the internet. Fortunately, I had some highly skilled and enthusiastic helpers, Rupert Wolfe Murray and Manuela Boghian, who inspired and helped me from the start. I would not have reached this stage without them. I am truly grateful. Richard Cross built the Poetrychangeslives.com website and provided advice beyond the mere technical with unfailing good humour. Design skills came from James Hutcheson and Edward Crossan for the pages and Helen Wyllie for the beautiful cover. Others who gave much needed advice and encouragement include Ingrid Christie, Peter Lindsay, Lara and Luca Wolfe Murray. Annabel Burn helped me with proof reading and Maryam Ghaffari helped me with her advice and enthusiasm. As a social media ingenu, I received huge help and support from Mark Baldwin who made great progress in transforming me from a technical dinosaur into a sort of 'ancient geek'.

Ever present and I hope, smiling in the shadows are my two old friends Bill W and Dr Bob, neither of whom I have met. Nevertheless I owe them a huge debt for the help that they have given to millions besides myself.

I have left until last my marvellous, erudite and sapient editor, Stephanie Wolfe Murray whose unfailing support, kindness and enthusiasm has kept me going throughout this process *–holy, fair and wise is she, the heavens such grace did lend her, that she might admired be.*

My heartfelt gratitude to you all.

Introduction

Poetry and history have always gone well together: history has often been recorded in verse and much poetry has been written about historical events. The story of Troy might be long forgotten if Homer had not immortalised it in verse. And likewise, Homer himself might be forgotten if Troy had not existed.

Historical facts, even those about kings and battles, can be dry reading but adding the poet's view can bring life and insight. The Hundred Years War becomes much more interesting if studied in conjunction with Shakespeare's play *King Henry V*.

It seemed odd to me that although history can be written in verse, and poems can be written about history, hardly any books exist that combine both historic facts with actual poems. It became my mission to create one and *Poetry Changes Lives* is the result.

I chose the title because poetry really did change my life, at different times in different ways. English poetry has been in my blood from the time I learned to read and I later grew to appreciate poetry from all over the world. I love it for its rhythms, its sounds and its insights but most of all I love the way poetry makes me feel. When I am low it gives me hope, when I am sad it makes me happy and when just bored, it gives me interest. By changing my feelings it changes my thoughts and actions and that is how it changes my life.

History's details are often more interesting to me than the main events. I would rather know Marie Antoinette's last words at the guillotine: "I am sorry Sir, I did not mean to put it there" (she trod on the executioner's foot) than the reasons for the French Revolution. But adding a poem that is in some way linked to this event adds yet another interest for me and I hope, for the reader.

Some poems have been too long to include in full and I must apologise for this. I hope that those wishing to read the full poem will be able to find it on the web or in a book without too much trouble.

The daily thought or reflection at the end of each poem is intended to help the reader to start in a positive frame of mind. I learnt the value of this in an alcohol rehab some years ago. The daily thought does not seek to promote any cause and no offence is intended to any person.

Christopher Burn

January 1st

The New Year officially begins today. We all want to make a good start to the year, a new beginning, but we don't always get it right.

Here is how Samuel Pepys began his in 1662: "Waking this morning out of my sleep on a sudden, I did with my elbow hit my wife a great blow over her face and nose, which waked her with pain, at which I was sorry, and to sleep again."

Pepys never lost his enthusiasm for life and nor should we, for life is too short to waste. We should seize each day. American poetess Sara Teasdale put it like this:

> Life has loveliness to sell,
> All beautiful and splendid things,
> Blue waves whitened on a cliff,
> Soaring fire that sways and sings,
> And children's faces looking up
> Holding wonder like a cup.
> Life has loveliness to sell,
> Music like a curve of gold,
> Scent of pine trees in the rain,
> Eyes that love you, arms that hold,
> And for your spirit's still delight,
> Holy thoughts that star the night.
> Spend all you have for loveliness,
> Buy it and never count the cost;
> For one white singing hour of peace
> Count many a year of strife well lost,
> And for a breath of ecstasy
> Give all you have been, or could be.

Today and all of this new year, I will try to live each day to the full, enjoying every moment that is given to me.

January 2nd

On this day in 1920, the author and academic Isaac Asimov was born. A brilliant thinker and leading science fiction writer, he was fascinated by change and its effects on our future. A Professor of biochemistry at Boston University, Asimov was a prolific writer and a brilliant lecturer. He wrote many textbooks on history and biochemistry as well as on literature. He loved to put a sci-fi slant on anything, including poetry. Here is the poem that he called 'The most remarkable example of science fiction poetry that has ever been written.'

It is, rather surprisingly, from *Locksley Hall* by Alfred Lord Tennyson:

For I dipped into the future, far as human eye could see,
Saw the vision of the world, and all the wonder that would be;
Saw the heavens fill with commerce, argosies of magic sails,
Pilots of the purple twilight, dropping down with costly bales;
Heard the heavens fill with shouting, and there rained a ghastly dew
From the nations' airy navies grappling in the central blue;
Far along the world-wide whisper of the south-wind rushing warm,
With the standards of the peoples plunging through the thunder-storm;
Till the war-drum throbbed no longer, and the battle-flags were furled
In the Parliament of man, the Federation of the world.

Today I reflect on how I view the world – that there are more things in heaven and earth than are dreamt of in our philosophy.

January 3rd

On this day in 106 BC the Roman Statesman Marcus Tullius Cicero was born. The surname Cicero means 'chickpea', probably because his family were dry food merchants and naming people in this way was the custom: for example, the well-known names Fabius, Lentulus, and Piso are the Latin names for bean, lentil and pea. An active politician, he was assassinated during the violent end of the Roman Republic.

Today's poem by Walt Whitman was written after another assassination – that of President Lincoln in 1865. Though nearly two thousand years after Cicero's death, the despair and sadness that it evoked were probably the same in both cases:

Captain! My Captain! Our fearful trip is done,
The ship has weather'd every rack, the prize we sought is won,
The port is near, the bells I hear, the people all exulting,
While follow eyes the steady keel, the vessel grim and daring;
But O heart! Heart! Heart!
O the bleeding drops of red,
Where on the deck my Captain lies,
Fallen cold and dead.

My Captain does not answer, his lips are pale and still,
My father does not feel my arm, he has no pulse nor will,
The ship is anchor'd safe and sound, its voyage closed and done,
From fearful trip the victor ship comes in with object won;
Exult O shores, and ring O bells!
But I with mournful tread,
Walk the deck my Captain lies,
Fallen cold and dead.

Today I will try to understand that great things can come out of terrible disasters.

January 4th

On this day in 1965 the poet Thomas Stearns (TS) Eliot died aged 76. A sickly child, born in St Louis, Missouri, he discovered poetry at an early age and travelled the world both to study (at the Sorbonne and Oxford) and to gain inspiration. London attracted him rather than the academic life in Oxford. He worked for some years in a bank before joining publishers Faber and Faber. Eliot knew many literary figures of the time such as Ezra Pound, James Joyce, WH Auden and Stephen Spender, many of whom he helped to publish. A quiet man and a heavy smoker, he died of emphysema.

Here is a poem about death and time, both themes that Eliot liked to use. This is by John Donne, *What if this present:*

> *What if this present were the world's last night?*
> *Marke in my heart, O Soule, where thou dost dwell,*
> *The picture of Christ crucified, and tell*
> *Whether that countenance can thee affright,*
> *Teares in his eyes quench the amazing light,*
> *Blood fills his frownes, which from his pierc'd head fell.*
> *And can that tongue adjudge thee into hell,*
> *Which pray'd forgivenesse for his foes fierce spight?*
> *No, no; but as in my idolatrie*
> *I said to all my profane mistresses,*
> *Beauty, of pity, foulenesse onely is*
> *A sign of rigour: so I say to thee,*
> *To wicked spirits are horrid shapes assign'd,*
> *This beauteous forme assures a piteous minde.*

Today I seek tolerance in myself for the shortcomings or insensitivities of others so that I can love the good qualities that they have.

January 5th

On this day in 1463 the French poet François Villon was banished from Paris. He was born in 1431, the year that Joan of Arc was burned to death. The bad boy of early French poetry, he killed a drunken priest and was imprisoned several times. Villon spent most of his life as a wandering ne'er do well; we have no record of him after 1463 and do not know when or how he died. His wonderfully direct poetry shows us what it was like to be alive in mediaeval Paris.

Here is part of his most famous poem which has been quoted countless times by other authors and songwriters, such as in the *Ballade des Dames du Temps Jadis (Song of the Ladies of Times Gone By):*

> *Tell me where, in which country*
> *Is Flora, the beautiful Roman;*
> *Archipiada, and Thaïs*
> *Who was her first cousin*
> *Echo, speaking when one makes noises*
> *over river or on pond*
> *Who had a beauty too much more than human?*
> *Oh, where are the snows of yesteryear!*
> *Where is the wise Heloise,*
> *For whom was castrated, and made a monk*
> *Pierre Abelard in Saint-Denis*
> *For his love he suffered this sentence.*
> *The queen Blanche, white as a lily*
> *Who sang with a Siren's voice*
> *Bertha of the Big Foot, Beatrix, Aelis;*
> *And Joan, the good woman from Lorraine*
> *Whom the English burned in Rouen ;*
> *Prince, do not ask me in the whole week*
> *Where they are – neither in this whole year,*
> *Lest I bring you back to this refrain –*
> *Oh, where are the snows of yesteryear!*

Today I will seek to love others not as I want them to be but as they really are.

January 6th

On this day in 1883 the Lebanese poet, painter and mystic writer Khalil Gibran was born. A Maronite Christian, Gibran believed in universal spirituality and was influenced by Islamic, Jewish and Baha'i thinking. His family moved to Boston when he was a child but he never became a US citizen. His writing, especially his book *The Prophet*, has been hugely influential and admirers as diverse as Carl Jung and Elvis Presley carried his books with them. Gibran's own life was not quite as tranquil as his writings imply; a gambler and an alcoholic, he died at the early age of 48 of cancer and cirrhosis of the liver. Nevertheless, he is the third most widely read author of all time. Here is part of one of his poems, *God*:

And after a thousand years I climbed the holy mountain and spoke unto God again, saying, 'Father, I am thy son. In pity and love thou hast given me birth, and through love and worship I shall inherit thy kingdom.'
And God made no answer, and like the mist that veils the distant ills he passed away.
And after a thousand years I climbed the sacred mountain and again spoke unto God, saying, 'My God, my aim and my fulfilment; I am thy yesterday and thou art my tomorrow. I am thy root in the earth and thou art my flower in the sky, and together we grow before the face of the sun.
Then God leaned over me, and in my ears whispered words of sweetness, and even as the sea that enfoldeth a brook that runneth down to her, he enfolded me.
And when I descended to the valleys and the plains, God was there also.

Today I reflect upon the universal spirituality of people whatever religion they may follow.

January 7th

On this day in 1326 King Edward II of England was deposed by forces led by his wife Isabella and her favourite, the exiled Roger de Mortimer. The son of the fearsome Edward I, the Hammer of the Scots, Edward had ruled for 20 years. He was perceived as weak and indecisive and tended to have favourites at court to whom he entrusted much power. Eventually his wife Isabella (known as the 'She-Wolf of France'), had had enough and joined Mortimer who was plotting to overthrow him. Edward was deposed in favour of his son Edward III and imprisoned at Berkeley Castle where he was later murdered. Mortimer was later executed for treason but Isabella was allowed to live on in comfort until she died 20 years later.

This poem is *The Female of the Species*, by Rudyard Kipling:

When the Himalayan peasant meets the he-bear in his pride,
He shouts to scare the monster, who will often turn aside.
But the she-bear thus accosted rends the peasant tooth and nail.
For the female of the species is more deadly than the male.
When Nag the basking cobra hears the careless foot of man,
He will sometimes wriggle sideways and avoid it if he can.
But his mate makes no such motion where she camps beside the trail.
For the female of the species is more deadly than the male.
When the early Jesuit fathers preached to Hurons and Choctaws,
They prayed to be delivered from the vengeance of the squaws.
Twas the women not the warriors, turned those stark enthusiasts
  pale.
For the female of the species is more deadly than the male.
Man's timid heart is bursting with the things he must not say,
For the Woman that God gave him isn't his to give away;
But when hunter meets with husbands each confirms the other's
  tale –
The female of the species is more deadly than the male.

Today I will try to no longer be a people pleaser and approval seeker but to have the strength and courage to be myself.

January 8th

On this day in 1902 the psychologist Carl Rogers was born. Rogers is considered one of the founding fathers of psychotherapy. Many of his concepts such as the 'unconditional positive regard' that a counsellor should give their client and the theory of communication between client and clinician, are in use today, as is his concept of the "Fully Functioning Person". Rogers was voted second to Sigmund Freud in a rating of the most effective clinical psychologists of all time.

Today's poem is from *The Garden of Proserpine* by Swinburne and talks of the kind of feelings that may lead us into therapy:

We are not sure of sorrow,
And joy was never sure;
To-day will die to-morrow;
Time stoops to no man's lure;
And love, grown faint and fretful,
With lips but half regretful
Sighs, and with eyes forgetful
Weeps that no loves endure.
From too much love of living,
From hope and fear set free,
We thank with brief thanksgiving

Whatever gods may be
That no life lives for ever;
That dead men rise up never;
That even the weariest river
Winds somewhere safe to sea.
Then star nor sun shall waken,
Nor any change of light:
Nor sound of waters shaken,
Nor any sound or sight:
Nor wintry leaves nor vernal,
Nor days nor things diurnal;
Only the sleep eternal
In an eternal night.

Today I will try to help people by giving them unconditional positive regard and not by telling them what to do.

January 9th

On this day 1776 Thomas Paine published *Common Sense*, a pamphlet that was a scathing attack on King George III's reign over the colonies and a call for complete independence. His pamphlets were hugely influential and read by every colonial patriot. As John Adams said, "Without the pen of the author of *Common Sense*, the sword of Washington would have been raised in vain."

Paine returned to Europe and lived in France during the 1790's where he wrote his famous work *The Rights of Man*. He took an active part in the revolution and, unusually for an Englishman, got elected to the French National Convention, where Robespierre regarded him as an enemy. Paine's last years were spent back in America where he fell out with many, including George Washington whom he accused of conspiring with Robespierre against him. He died in New York; sadly the funeral of the man who had influenced so many was attended by just six people.

Here is his poem, *Lines Extempore:*

Quick as the lightning's vivid flash
The poet's eye o'er Europe rolls;
Sees battles rage, hears tempests crash,
And dims at horror's threatening scowls –
Marks ambition's ruthless king,
With crimson'd banners scathe the globe,
While trailing after conquest's wing,
Man's festering wounds his demons probe.
Palled with streams of reeking gore –
That stain the proud imperial day;
He turns to view the Western shore,
Where freedom holds her boundless sway.
'Tis here her sage triumphant sways
An empire in the people's love,
'Tis here the sovereign will obeys
No King but Him who rules above.

Today I will try to live my life using common sense.

January 10th

On this day in 49 BC Julius Caesar and his army crossed the Rubicon (it was illegal for a general to bring an army into Italy – the River Rubicon was the boundary line). Fresh from his conquests in Germany, Gaul and Britain, Caesar refused the senate's order to resign his military commission. The resulting civil war left him victorious and he assumed control of the state, bringing in a number of reforms.

However his enemies were plotting and on the Ides of March in 44 BC he was assassinated in the Senate and war followed again, resulting in the rise of his nominated heir Octavian, who became the first emperor, taking the name Augustus. Besides being a brilliant general and a skilled politician, Caesar left his own written accounts of his campaigns.

Here is a poem by Kipling, the poet of a later empire:

> Cities and Thrones and Powers
> Stand in Time's eye,
> Almost as long as flowers,
> Which daily die:
> But, as new buds put forth
> To glad new men,
> Out of the spent and unconsidered Earth,
> The Cities rise again.
> So Time that is o'er-kind
> To all that be,
> Ordains us e'en as blind,
> As bold as she:
> That in our very death,
> And burial sure,
> Shadow to shadow, well persuaded, saith,
> "See how our works endure!"

Today I marvel at the fame of a man whose name became synonymous with King. I am grateful to be anonymous.

January 11th

On this day in 2008 the New Zealand mountaineer Edmund Hillary died aged 88. He will always be remembered for the 1952 conquest of Everest, the world's highest mountain, with Sherpa Tenzing.

Both were clearly big achievers but they were also humble men; Hillary photographed Tenzing at the summit but then indicated that he did not want to be photographed himself. Tenzing left behind some chocolates as a gift for the gods, Hillary left a small wooden cross that had been given to expedition leader Sir John Hunt by the abbot of Ampleforth Abbey, Yorkshire. For the rest of his life Hillary continued exploration and visited both the North and South poles. He also worked tirelessly to improve the lot of the Nepalese, especially the Sherpas. Following his death he was given a state funeral. In Nepal he is still treated like a god.

Today's poem by Christina Rossetti is called, suitably for Hillary, *Up-Hill*:

Does the road wind up-hill all the way?
  Yes, to the very end.
Will the day's journey take the whole long day?
  From morn to night, my friend.
But is there for the night a resting-place?
  A roof for when the slow dark hours begin.
May not the darkness hide it from my face?
  You cannot miss that inn.
Shall I meet other wayfarers at night?
  Those who have gone before.
Then must I knock, or call when just in sight?
  They will not keep you standing at that door.
Shall I find comfort, travel-sore and weak?
  Of labour you shall find the sum.
Will there be beds for me and all who seek?
  Yea, beds for all who come.

Today I know that happiness comes from a successful journey.

January 12th

On this day in 1876 the novelist Jack London was born in San Francisco. Famous for his tales of adventure and struggles against adversity such as *White Fang, The Call of the Wild* and *The Sea Wolf,* London often wrote from personal experience as a hobo, a sailor, a jailbird, an oyster pirate and a miner in the Klondike gold rush. His work had great popularity and he was known as a man who liked to live life to the full.

Here is his 'credo' that he published with his short stories: "I would rather be ashes than dust! I would rather that my spark should burn out in a brilliant blaze than it should be stifled by dry-rot. I would rather be a superb meteor, every atom of me in magnificent glow, than a sleepy and permanent planet. The function of man is to live, not to exist. I shall not waste my days in trying to prolong them. I shall use my time." Besides writing novels he also wrote poetry.

> Here is one entitled George Sterling:
> I saw a man open an iris petal.
> He ran his finger underneath the edge,
> unfolded it, and smoothed it out a little,
> not as one guilty of a sacrilege –
> because he knew flowers, and understood
> that what he did would maybe help them grow –
> though for a moment he was almost God.
> Alone as we are, growing is so slow.
> I think of one who tried like that to unfold
> the margin of his life where it was curled,
> to see into the shadows shot with gold
> that lie in iris hues about the world.
> Because he dared to touch the sacred rim,
> does God resent this eagerness in him?

Today I reflect on the freedom that comes from the surrender of one's will to a higher power.

January 13th

On this day in 1941 the author James Joyce died in Zurich. Regularly considered one of the most influential writers of the 20th century, Joyce grew up in Dublin in a family damaged by his father's drinking. A brilliant student, though feckless with money and a heavy drinker, he went to live in Europe with his long-time girlfriend Norah Barnacle, mostly in Trieste, Zurich and then Paris where, over a number of years, he wrote his great work *Ulysses*. Joyce was also an accomplished pianist and guitar player as well as a poet of merit. He was sometimes a diffident man for all his scholarship and described himself to Carl Jung as 'A man of small virtue, inclined to extravagance and alcoholism'. His first short poems were published under the title *Chamber Music* which, he joked, was the sound of urine hitting a chamber pot.

Here is an example:

> *Who goes amid the green wood*
> *With springtide all adorning her?*
> *Who goes amid the merry green wood*
> *To make it merrier?*
> *Who passes in the sunlight*
> *By ways that know the light footfall?*
> *Who passes in the sweet sunlight*
> *With mien so virginal?*
> *The ways of all the woodland*
> *Gleam with a soft and golden fire –*
> *For whom does all the sunny woodland*
> *Carry so brave attire?*
> *O, it is for my true love*
> *The woods their rich apparel wear –*
> *O, it is for my own true love,*
> *That is so young and fair.*

Today I give thanks for my health and ask that I be kept free from the scourge of alcoholism.

January 14th

On this day in 1875 the French physician, missionary, philosopher and musician Albert Schweitzer was born. An expert pianist and organist, he became an authority on the building and restoration of historic church organs. However, at the age of thirty, he decided that he would give himself to humanity, with Jesus serving as his example. He therefore studied both medicine and theology with the idea of becoming a missionary and was eventually able to secure backing for the establishment of a hospital in Gabon, West Africa.

In 1913 he and his wife and son departed for Africa and established the famous hospital at Lambaréné in Gabon. It still exists today. This became the main focus of his life's work until he died there in 1965. In 1952 he received the Nobel Peace Prize for his philosophical work *Reverence for Life*. Schweitzer was a friend of Albert Einstein and Bertrand Russell and active in promoting nuclear disarmament and world peace. He also loved animals, whom he felt should be respected more.

He wrote *A Prayer for Animals*:

> *Hear our humble prayer, O God,*
> *For our friends the animals,*
> *Especially for those who are suffering;*
> *For any that are hunted or lost*
> *Or deserted or frightened or hungry;*
> *For all that must be put to sleep.*
> *We entreat for them all Thy mercy and pity,*
> *And for those who deal with them*
> *We ask a heart of compassion*
> *And gentle hands and kindly words.*
> *Make us be true friends to animals*
> *And so to share the blessings of the merciful.*

Today I reflect on the example of Albert Schweitzer, who has been a force for good in the world.

January 15th

On this day in 1886 Colonel John Pemberton registered the Pemberton Medicine Company in Atlanta, Georgia which would later become the Coca-Cola Company. Pemberton was a civil war veteran who had been wounded and subsequently became addicted to morphine.

He was looking for a substitute medicine. Coca-Cola was initially sold for five cents a glass at soda fountains, then highly popular in America. The formula for the drink called for five ounces of coca leaf per gallon of syrup, a significant dose of what was, effectively, cocaine – an estimated nine milligrams per glass. In 1903, this substance was removed.

Daily servings of the drink are now estimated to be 1.9 billion. Coca-Cola has been drunk in outer space and today the word is considered the second most widely understood throughout the world (the first is 'ok'). That's a long way from an average five servings a day in an Atlanta drugstore in 1886.

Today's poem is by William Butler Yeats, entitled *A Drinking Song*:

> *Wine comes in at the mouth*
> *And love comes in at the eye;*
> *That's all we shall know for truth*
> *Before we grow old and die.*
> *I lift the glass to my mouth,*
> *I look at you, and I sigh.*

I look at the world and the stranglehold that big business sometimes seems to have on people and tell myself to accept the things I cannot change and to be grateful for the things I have. Like Coca-Cola.

January 16th

On this day in 1793 the French King Louis XVI was sentenced to death by the National Convention in Paris. Louis seems to have been deluded into thinking that the people wanted him to stay on as king.

His fatal indecision rendered him incapable of responding to events. Indeed it seems to have been the proactive, though inexperienced, Marie Antoinette who tried to steer the family through their last desperate months. It was all to no avail and she followed him to the scaffold nine months later. Louis conducted himself well on the day of his execution and died bravely – the king who had been despised and disliked for his weakness finally gained the people's respect.

Today's poem is by DH Lawrence, *A Sane Revolution*:

> *If you make a revolution, make it for fun,*
> *Don't make it in ghastly seriousness,*
> *Don't do it in deadly earnest, do it for fun.*
> *Don't do it because you hate people,*
> *Do it just to spit in their eye.*
> *Don't do it for the money,*
> *Do it and be damned to the money.*
> *Don't do it for equality,*
> *Do it because we've got too much equality*
> *And it would be fun to upset the apple-cart*
> *And see which way the apples would go a-rolling.*
> *Don't do it for the working classes.*
> *Do it so that we can all of us be little aristocracies on our own*
> *And kick our heels like jolly escaped asses.*
> *Don't do it, anyhow, for international Labour.*
> *Labour is the one thing a man has had too much of.*
> *Let's abolish labour, let's have done with labouring!*
> *Work can be fun, and men can enjoy it; then it's not labour.*
> *Let's have it so! Let's make a revolution for fun!*

Today I will try to conduct myself bravely in everything.

January 17th

On this day in 1706 the American writer, politician, scientist and diplomat Benjamin Franklin was born. Franklin was hugely industrious and inventive. He was a successful newspaper publisher and also worked on inventions involving electricity – he produced the first lightning rod.

He was politically active and his communication skills were so good that he seems to have been involved in talks with the British government before the War of Independence as well as being ambassador to France where he spent several years. Franklin was interested in education and helped to found the University of Pennsylvania.

Twenty thousand people came to his funeral in 1790. This is the epitaph that he wrote for himself : The Body of B. Franklin Printer; Like the Cover of an old Book, Its Contents torn out, and stript of its Lettering and Gilding, Lies here, Food for Worms. But the Work shall not be wholly lost: For it will, as he believ'd, appear once more, In a new & more perfect Edition, Corrected and Amended By the Author. Franklin was an accomplished writer and his autobiography makes for good reading.

His poems reflect his playful, less serious side. Here is one, *Equivocation*:

> Some have learn't many tricks of sly evasion,
> Instead of truth they use equivocation,
> And eke it out with mental reservation,
> Which, to good men, is an abomination.
> Our smith of late most wonderfully swore,
> That whilst he breathed he would drink no more,
> But since, I know his meaning, for I think,
> He meant he would not breathe whilst he did drink.

Today I will strive to keep things simple and not complicate my life unnecessarily by trying to do things that do not suit me.

January 18th

On this day in 1882 the author and journalist AA Milne was born. He found the success of the Pooh Bear stories increasingly annoying, though he could do nothing about it except keep writing.

A hundred years later, the stories, many now in cartoon form, are still a huge hit with children and adults all over the world. Milne started writing them for his child Christopher Robin, using the nursery toys as characters. Though he continued to write other stories and plays, their success was negligible – all that the public wanted from him was nursery talk. Milne died of a stroke in 1956, still regretting that he was not taken more seriously.

This poem (extract) by Edward Lear will be equally familiar to many, *The Owl and the Pussy-Cat*:

> *The Owl and the Pussy-cat went to sea*
> *In a beautiful pea-green boat,*
> *They took some honey, and plenty of money,*
> *Wrapped up in a five-pound note.*
> *The Owl looked up to the stars above,*
> *And sang to a small guitar,*
> *"O lovely Pussy! O Pussy, my love,*
> *What a beautiful Pussy you are,*
> *What a beautiful Pussy you are!*
> *Pussy said to the Owl, "You elegant fowl!*
> *How charmingly sweet you sing! They dined on mince, and slices of quince,*
> *Which they ate with a runcible spoon;*
> *And hand in hand, on the edge of the sand,*
> *They danced by the light of the moon,*
> *They danced by the light of the moon.*

Today, though I am grateful for childish things, I understand that I am an adult and must deal with the real world.

January 19th

On this day in 1809 the novelist Edgar Allan Poe was born. Although now well-known, he was beset for most of his life with financial problems, perhaps caused by drink. He worked for several newspapers and magazines but struggled to make a living as a writer. Eventually some of his stories and poetry gained recognition, but by then his private life had started to deteriorate – his marriage to his 13-year-old cousin ended when she died of consumption aged 22.

His drinking became worse; he died in Baltimore aged 40, of causes unknown, though delirium tremens or rabies was suspected. The man whose own life was hard to understand engendered a whole new genre of writing crime fiction that inspired others such as Sir Arthur Conan Doyle, Jules Verne and Agatha Christie.

Some of his poetry was very popular. This example, a poem called *Eldorado* was written in response to the California gold rush:

Gaily bedight,
A gallant knight,
In sunshine and in shadow,
Had journeyed long,
Singing a song,
In search of Eldorado.
But he grew old –
This knight so bold –
And o'er his heart a shadow
Fell as he found
No spot of ground
That looked like Eldorado.

And, as his strength
Failed him at length,
He met a pilgrim shadow –
"Shadow," said he,
"Where can it be –
This land of Eldorado?"

Today I shall set achievable goals.

January 20th

On this day in 1961 the inauguration of President John F Kennedy took place in Washington DC. The 86 year old poet Robert Frost recited some of his poetry from memory (the sun was in his eyes so he could not read it). The inauguration finished and Kennedy's thousand days in office began.

One of his favourite poems was this one by Alan Seeger, which has a grim prophetic ring to it:

> I have a rendezvous with Death
> At some disputed barricade,
> When Spring comes back with rustling shade
> And apple-blossoms fill the air –
> I have a rendezvous with Death
> When Spring brings back blue days and fair.
> It may be he shall take my hand
> And lead me into his dark land
> And close my eyes and quench my breath –
> It may be I shall pass him still.
> I have a rendezvous with Death
> On some scarred slope of battered hill,
> When Spring comes round again this year
> And the first meadow-flowers appear.
> God knows 'twere better to be deep
> Pillowed in silk and scented down,
> Where hushed awakenings are dear
> But I've a rendezvous with Death
> At midnight in some flaming town,
> When Spring trips north again this year,
> And I to my pledged word am true,
> I shall not fail that rendezvous.

Today I reflect on the future with faith in the inherent goodness of mankind.

January 21st

On this day in 1905 the French fashion designer Christian Dior was born. Dior grew up in the Normandy seaside town of Granville-sur-Mer but was soon working in Paris for a number of well-known fashion designers, including Balmain and Patou. During the Second World War, he was forced to design dresses for Nazi wives while his sister was fighting in the Resistance and later imprisoned at Ravensbruck concentration camp.

After the war he started his own fashion house which he quickly built up into a global brand. The name of Dior became synonymous with the best in fashion. He is most remembered for his 'New Look' which brought back longer and fuller skirts; these used more material and initially upset women who had been used to wearing skimpy clothes and short skirts, necessitated by wartime shortages of dress material. Dior died aged 52 while on holiday in Italy. The world lost a great designer, but the name lives on.

Perhaps Dior knew this famous poem by 17th century poet Robert Herrick:

When as in silks my Julia goes
Then, then (methinks) how sweetly flows
That liquefaction of her clothes.
Next when I cast my eyes and see
That brave vibration each way free
Oh how that glittering taketh me.

Today I give thanks for a sharpened sense of reality that I get from reflection and understanding of myself.

January 22nd

On this day in 1788 George Gordon Byron, known as Lord Byron, was born. 'Mad, bad and dangerous to know' was the famous summation of Lady Caroline Lamb.

Most literature about Byron tends to list people of both sexes whom he met, followed by the words 'with whom he had an affair'. Such people included school friends at Harrow, servant girls, his close relations, society ladies, the poet Shelley, other men's wives and 'When nine years old at his mother's house a free Scotch girl called Mary Gray, who used to come to bed to him and play tricks with his person.' He died in Greece aged 36, an adventurer to the last.

This piece is said to have been inspired by meeting and falling in love with a beautiful widow at a ball. Her black dress was set with spangles, *She Walks in Beauty*:

> She walks in beauty, like the night
>   Of cloudless climes and starry skies;
> And all that's best of dark and bright
>   Meet in her aspect and her eyes;
> Thus mellowed to that tender light
>   Which heaven to gaudy day denies.
> One shade the more, one ray the less,
>   Had half impaired the nameless grace
> Which waves in every raven tress,
>   Or softly lightens o'er her face;
> Where thoughts serenely sweet express,
>   How pure, how dear their dwelling-place.
> And on that cheek, and o'er that brow,
>   So soft, so calm, yet eloquent,
> The smiles that win, the tints that glow,
>   But tell of days in goodness spent,
> A mind at peace with all below,
>   A heart whose love is innocent!

Today I reflect on the good in people rather than their faults.

January 23rd

On this day in 1832 the French painter Edouard Manet was born. A major influence on later artists, Manet's work represents the transition from Realism to Impressionism. Born into a well to do Parisian family, he could afford to travel and study the masters whose work he greatly admired and often paraphrased; for example, his famous painting *Le Déjeuner sur l'Herbe* follows the composition of a Raphael drawing.

His *Olympia* is reminiscent of Goya's *Naked Maja*. Much of his work contains homage to the old masters, especially Franz Hals, Velasquez and Goya. Manet knew almost everyone in the Paris art world – Degas, Monet, Pisarro, Cezanne and Renoir and also the writers Emile Zola, Stephan Mallarmé and Charles Baudelaire.

It seems that even such an array as these could not stop him from wandering off the path of righteousness. He died of complications from syphilis at the age of 51.

Today's poem is by Christopher Marlowe. It springs to mind when looking at *Le Déjeuner sur l'Herbe*:

> *but we will leave this paltry land*
> *And sail from hence to Greece, to lovely Greece.*
> *I'll be thy Jason, thou my golden fleece.*
> *Where painted carpets o'er the meads are hurled,*
> *And Bacchus' vineyards overspread the world,*
> *Where woods and forests go in goodly green,*
> *I'll be Adonis: thou shalt be Love's Queen.*
> *The meads, the orchards, and the primrose lanes,*
> *Instead of sedge and reed, bear sugar canes.*
> *Thou in those groves, by Dis above,*
> *Shalt live with me, and be my love.*

Today I am grateful for the endless and uncomplicated pleasure that comes from viewing great works of art.

January 24th

On this day in 1965 Winston Churchill died in London, aged 90. Throughout his extraordinary life, Churchill experienced a huge variety of situations, including being under fire many times. As a soldier, war correspondent, member of parliament and statesman, he travelled the world meeting kings, presidents and dictators.

On one occasion he nearly met his arch enemy, Adolf Hitler, as recounted in his book *The Gathering Storm*. Churchill is also remarkable for his many hobbies which included painting, butterfly breeding and bricklaying. He is a national hero in a similar way to Sir Francis Drake, who famously defeated the Spanish Armada in 1588.

The sentiments behind Henry Newbolt's poem *Drake's Drum* could apply to Churchill. Here is the first stanza:

> Drake he's in his hammock an' a thousand mile away,
>   (Capten, art tha sleepin' there below?)
> Slung atween the round shot in Nombre Dios Bay,
>   An' dreamin' arl the time o' Plymouth Hoe.
> Yarnder lumes the island, yarnder lie the ships,
>   Wi' sailor lads a-dancin' heel-an'-toe,
> An' the shore-lights flashin', an' the night-tide dashin'
>   He sees it arl so plainly as he saw it long ago.
> Drake he was a Devon man, an' ruled the Devon seas,
>   (Capten, art tha sleepin' there below?),
> Rovin' tho' his death fell, he went wi' heart at ease,
>   An' dreamin' arl the time o' Plymouth Hoe,
> "Take my drum to England, hang it by the shore,
>   Strike it when your powder's runnin' low;
> If the Dons sight Devon, I'll quit the port o' Heaven,
>   An' drum them up the Channel as we drummed them long ago."

Today I am grateful for the courage and determination of all great men.

January 25th

On this day in 1759 the Scottish poet Robert Burns was born. A Customs Officer, he travelled around Scotland and enjoyed dalliance with many pretty girls. He is known to have fathered 12 children and is estimated to have over six hundred living descendants.

Burns was a great egalitarian who supported the French Revolution, as is shown in part of his famous poem, *A Man's a Man for A'That*:

> *Is there for honest Poverty*
> *That hings his head, an' a' that;*
> *The coward slave, we pass him by,*
> *We dare be poor for a' that!*
> *For a' that, an' a' that.*
> *Our toils obscure an' a' that,*
> *The rank is but the guinea's stamp,*
> *The Man's the gowd for a' that.*
> *Then let us pray that come it may,*
> *(As come it will for a' that,)*
> *That Sense and Worth, o'er a' the earth,*
> *Shall bear the gree, an' a' that.*
> *For a' that, an' a' that,*
> *It's coming yet for a' that,*
> *That Man to Man, the world o'er,*
> *Shall brothers be for a' that.*

Burns died in 1796. His strong views found favour with Communist regimes in later years, and he is still highly popular in Russia.

Today I will reflect on the egalitarian views of 'The Scottish Bard', and treat all people as equals.

January 26th

On this day in 1849 the English poet Thomas Lovell Beddoes poisoned himself in Basel, Switzerland, aged 45. Beddoes grew up in Bristol and was a brilliant scholar, becoming a doctor of medicine.

He became obsessed with death and devoted much of his time to seeking proof of the physical existence of the human spirit. He seems to have become progressively more deranged and alcoholic but nevertheless managed to write some of the most hauntingly and uniquely beautiful poetry of the 19th century, much of it only appreciated after his death.

Here is his *Wulfram's Dirge*:

> If thou wilt ease thine heart
> Of love and all its smart,
>   Then sleep, dear, sleep;
> And not a sorrow
> Hang any tear on your eye-lashes;
>   Lie still and deep,
> Sad soul, until the sea-wave washes
> The rim o' the sun to-morrow,
>   In eastern sky.
> But wilt thou cure thine heart
> Of love and all its smart,
>   Then die, dear, die;
> 'Tis deeper, sweeter,
>   Than on a rose-bank to lie dreaming
>   With folded eye;
>   And there alone, amid the beaming
> Of Love's stars, thou'lt meet her
>   In eastern sky.

Today I ask that I will learn to appreciate and enjoy life and to be able to manage life's difficulties in a positive way.

January 27th

On this day in 1756 Wolfgang Amadeus Mozart was born in Salzburg. His loving father quickly realised that Wolfgang and his sister were exceptionally talented at music, and as early as 1762 (when his son was only six) he started taking them on concert tours to show off their skills. From Munich they went to Vienna to the court of the Holy Roman Emperor, who was delighted with their performances. Here, both children were allowed to play with the Hapsburg children, including the seven year old Marie Antoinette, future Queen of France.

The story goes that young Mozart slipped and fell on the polished floor. Marie Antoinette, who was almost exactly the boy's age, caught him. He kissed her and told her "I'll marry you some day." They never met again. Mozart died aged 35, in December 1791 – Marie Antoinette went to the guillotine in 1793.

Today's poem is about music, from Shakespeare's *Twelfth Night*:

> If music be the food of love, play on;
> Give me excess of it, that, surfeiting,
> The appetite may sicken, and so die.
> That strain again! It had a dying fall:
> O, it came o'er my ear like the sweet sound,
> That breathes upon a bank of violets,
> Stealing and giving odour! Enough; no more:
> 'Tis not so sweet now as it was before.
> O spirit of love! How quick and fresh art thou,
> That, notwithstanding thy capacity
> Receiveth as the sea, nought enters there,
> Of what validity and pitch soe'er,
> But falls into abatement and low price,
> Even in a minute: so full of shapes is fancy
> That it alone is high fantastical.

Today I give thanks for opportunities given to me to learn from others.

January 28th

On this day in 1813 Jane Austen's novel *Pride and Prejudice* was published. Like all her work, it was read aloud to her family most evenings as she was writing it. The themes of all Jane's writing are morality, respectability and the need for young women to find husbands. Though she died two years after the Battle of Waterloo, her characters seemed blissfully unaware of the upheavals and carnage going on in Europe at the time.

Today's poem, by Ernest Dowson, is about a special kind of faithfulness – *Non sum qualis eram bonae sub regno Cynarae*:

> Last night, ah, yesternight, betwixt her lips and mine
> There fell thy shadow, Cynara! Thy breath was shed
> Upon my soul between the kisses and the wine;
> And I was desolate and sick of an old passion,
>   Yea, I was desolate and bowed my head:
> I have been faithful to thee, Cynara! In my fashion.
> I have forgot much, Cynara! Gone with the wind,
> Flung roses, roses riotously with the throng,
> Dancing, to put thy pale, lost lilies out of mind,
> But I was desolate and sick of an old passion,
>   Yea, all the time, because the dance was long:
> I have been faithful to thee, Cynara! In my fashion.
> I cried for madder music and for stronger wine,
> But when the feast is finished and the lamps expire,
> Then falls thy shadow, Cynara! The night is thine;
> And I am desolate and sick of an old passion,
>   Yea, hungry for the lips of my desire:
> I have been faithful to thee Cynara! In my fashion.

Today I give thanks for the virtues of faithfulness and loyalty that mean so much as we grow older and wiser.

January 29th

On this day in 1595 the first performance of Shakespeare's *Romeo and Juliet* took place. This tale of teenage love, violence and death is the most sexually charged of all Shakespeare's plays, which may account for its popularity and explain why it has been filmed so many times. It contains some of the most beautiful lines that the bard ever wrote.

If the play was simply a story of adolescent romance, it would not have been so well remembered. As always, Shakespeare has other messages to give. Take Romeo for example – he is not just a hormonal teenager helplessly driven by his emotions, but a youth who grows up and acts decisively, once his friend Mercutio has been killed. In other words, love turns young men into wimps and that wasn't good, either in 14th century Verona or in 16th century London where young men had to be fighters to survive.

Not everyone liked the play. Diarist Samuel Pepys wrote in 1662: "It is a play of itself the worst that I ever heard in my life." Luckily, most people did not agree.

Here are some of the most famous lines in the play, if not in all literature:

> But, soft! What light through yonder window breaks?
> It is the east, and Juliet is the sun.
> Arise, fair sun, and kill the envious moon,
> Who is already sick and pale with grief,
> That thou, her maid, art far more fair than she.
> Be not her maid, since she is envious;
> Her vestal livery is but sick and green
> And none but fools do wear it; cast it off.
> It is my lady, O, it is my love!
> Oh, that she knew she were!

Today I reflect upon spirituality and the need to understand emotions rather than to be driven by them from day to day.

January 30th

On this day in 1649 King Charles I of England was beheaded at Whitehall Palace. It was a cold day and Charles wore two shirts so that the people might not see him shiver. His head was severed in one blow whereupon, in the words of one observer: "a groan, as I never heard before and desire I may never hear again" arose from the assembled crowd.

Later, the head was sewn back on and the body placed in a lead coffin. Oliver Cromwell, the man most responsible for the regicidal deed, visited the coffin and was heard to murmur the words "a cruel necessity". Charles' arrogance and belief in his divine right to rule had made him an impossible monarch, but his execution and the manner in which he conducted himself during it, turned him into a royal martyr.

The poet Andrew Marvell described the terrible event:

> He nothing common did or mean
> Upon that memorable scene:
> But with his keener eye
> The axe's edge did try.
> Nor called the gods with vulgar spite
> To vindicate his helpless right,
> But bowed his comely head
> Down as upon a bed.

Charles did not want any revenge taken for his death. However, following the restoration in 1660, his son Charles II pursued a relentless quest to bring the regicides (the 59 signatories to his father's death warrant) to justice. Eventually, 19 were executed and a further 19 were imprisoned.

Today I will reflect on forgiveness towards those that do me harm.

January 31st

On this day in 1923 the American author Norman Mailer was born. Mailer was one of a group of writers that included Hunter S. Thompson, Tom Wolfe, Gore Vidal and Truman Capote who had strong opinions and were prepared to act them out.

They were a godsend to TV presenters at a time when public inertia was widespread. Mailer was often to be found on the screen, belligerent and well refreshed, arguing on a variety of subjects and often responding physically to emphasise a point. On one famous occasion, Mailer head butted Vidal on live TV. His relationships were often stormy and he stabbed one of his wives with a penknife, earning himself the soubriquet 'Mailer the Impaler'. His first novel, *The Naked and the Dead* was a best seller as were several others and he won two Pulitzer Prizes.

Today's poem is by JK Stephen who mocked the literary styles of his day:

Will there never come a season
Which shall rid us from the curse
Of a prose which knows no reason
And an unmelodious verse:
When the world shall cease to wonder
At the genius of an Ass,
And a boy's eccentric blunder
Shall not bring success to pass:
When mankind shall be delivered
From the clash of magazines,
And the inkstand shall be shivered
Into countless smithereens:
When there stands a muzzled stripling,
Mute, beside a muzzled bore:
When the Rudyards cease from Kipling
And the Haggards Ride no more.

Today I reflect on aggression, but will respect all people as my brothers and sisters.

February 1st

On this day in 1903 the American poet Langston Hughes was born. Hughes was of mixed race and was highly influential in the Harlem Renaissance. Besides writing novels he wrote jazz poetry and considered himself to be a spokesman for the black working class.

He travelled a lot, especially to the Soviet Union where his work was seen as compatible with Communist ideology. Hughes was ahead of his time in his pride at being a Negro when racial equality was a dream, barely considered by many Americans.

This poem by Thomas Lovell Beddoes is about dreams, *Dream-Pedlary*:

> *If there were dreams to sell,*
> * What would you buy?*
> *Some cost a passing bell;*
> * Some a light sigh,*
> *That shakes from Life's fresh crown*
> *Only a rose-leaf down.*
> *If there were dreams to sell,*
> *Merry and sad to tell,*
> *And the crier rang the bell,*
> * What would you buy?*
> *A cottage lone and still,*
> * With bowers nigh,*
> *Shadowy, my woes to still,*
> * Until I die.*
> *Such pearl from Life's fresh crown*
> *Fain would I shake me down.*
> *Were dreams to have at will,*
> *This would best heal my ill,*
> * This would I buy.*

Today I reflect on equality for all, and expect progress not perfection.

February 2nd

On this day in 1846 the French journalist and poet Theophile Gautier wrote an account of his experiences at Club des Hashischins (Club of the Hashish-Eaters) a Parisian group dedicated to the exploration of drug-induced experiences. Members included Victor Hugo, Alexandre Dumas, Honoré de Balzac, Eugene Delacroix and Charles Baudelaire. The club had been started by Dr Jacques Joseph Moreau for mainly scientific research purposes but probably some of the attenders were 'only there for the gear.' Members dressed up in Arab costume and took the drug mainly as a syrup, with coffee.

It seems to have been Baudelaire, author of *Les Fleurs du Mal* and a known drug user, who derived most insight into the effects of cannabis. He believed that, more than the alcohol drinker, the hashish user was likely to suffer psychological problems, a view held by many professionals today.

Here is one of Gautier's poems entitled, rather aptly, *Smoke*:

> *Over there, trees are sheltering*
> *A hunchedback hut . . . A slum, no more . . .*
> *Roof askew, walls and wainscoting*
> *Falling away . . . Moss hides the door.*
> *Only one shutter, hanging . . . But*
> *Seeping over the windowsill,*
> *Like frosted breath, proof that this hut,*
> *This slum, is living, breathing still*
> *Corkscrew of smoke . . . A wisp of blue*
> *Escapes the hovel, whose soul it is . . .*
> *Rises to God himself, and who*
> *Receives the news and makes it his.*

Today I am grateful that my life is not affected by mood altering drugs and I will strive to ensure that it will remain so.

February 3rd

On this day in 1959 the American singer Buddy Holly was killed in a plane crash. It was the 'day the music died' for thousands of fans. Musicians killed in plane crashes since then include Otis Redding, Lynyrd Skynyrd band members, John Denver, Jim Reeves and Patsy Cline. There have been many other fatal accidents involving cars, boats and motor bikes not to mention shootings, suicides and drownings. Singers and musicians seem to have somehow evolved into people who live dangerously or who are, at any rate, highly accident prone.

The Buddy Holly disaster was immortalised by Don MacLean in his song *American Pie*; the fairy-tale of pop stardom suddenly developed a darker side. At times like that, it can help to go back to basics and for me that often means John Donne.

I really like his *Death Be Not Proud*:

> Death be not proud, though some have called thee
> Mighty and dreadful, for, thou art not so,
> For, those, whom thou think'st, thou dost overthrow,
> Die not, poore death, nor yet canst thou kill me.
> From rest and sleepe, which but thy pictures bee,
> Much pleasure, then from thee, much more must flow,
> And soonest our bestmen with thee doe goe,
>
> Rest of their bones, and soules deliverie.
> Thou art slave to Fate, Chance, kings, and desperate men,
> And dost with poyson, warre, and sicknesse dwell,
> And poppie, or charmes can make us sleepe as well,
> And better then thy stroake; why swell'st thou then;
> One short sleepe past, wee wake eternally,
> And death shall be no more; death, thou shalt die.

Today I remember those who have died young for whatever reason. I will remember, like John Donne, that 'one short sleep past, we wake eternally'.

February 4th

On this day in 1906 the cleric, theologian and anti-Nazi pacifist Dietrich Bonhoeffer was born into a large and loving family in Germany. With the rise to power of the Nazis, he found himself under pressure to switch from the intellectual to the practical side of Christianity. Twice in the 1930s he left Germany on the offer of work in safer countries but chose to return because his conscience told him to. He became an active opponent of the regime and was involved in the German resistance movement.

In the later stages of the war he was involved in the plot to assassinate Hitler in 1944 and was imprisoned. In 1945 he was tried and executed only weeks before the end of the war. Bonhoeffer remains today a shining example of a man prepared to listen to his conscience and to choose to stand up for his beliefs, whatever the cost.

Today's poem, *To Be a Pilgrim*, is by John Bunyan, a good choice for a very brave man:

Who would true Valour see
Let him come hither;
One here will Constant be,
Come Wind, come Weather.
There's no Discouragement,
Shall make him once Relent,
His first avow'd Intent,
To be a Pilgrim.
Who so beset him round,
With dismal Storys,
Do but themselves Confound;
His Strength the more is.
No Lyon can him fright,

He'll with a Gyant Fight,
But he will have a right,
To be a Pilgrim.
Hobgoblin, nor foul Fiend,
Can daunt his Spirit:
He knows, he at the end,
Shall Life Inherit.
Then Fancies fly away,
He'll fear not what men say,
He'll labour Night and Day,
To be a Pilgrim.

Today I give thanks for all brave men and women who stand up and fight against the powers of evil.

February 5th

On this day in 1914 the author William Burroughs was born. The son of wealthy parents, Burroughs was one of the group of enfants terribles of post war American letters who became known as the Beat Generation. Burroughs developed a heroin addiction as a student and never successfully overcame it. His peculiar disjointed writing perhaps reflects this.

He is best known for his prose work *Naked Lunch* which is basically a series of chapters mostly unconnected, that Burroughs said could be read in any order. It was the subject of an obscenity trial and banned in some US states. Burroughs also popularised the cut-up poetry technique whereby existing texts are cut up and rearranged to form new works. In one example (*Fear and the Monkey*), Burroughs has taken a poem by English writer Denton Welch and added "a pinch of Rimbaud, a dash of St-John Perse, an oblique reference to Toby Tyler with the Circus, and the death of his pet monkey."

Here is an anonymous taste of cut-up poetry that includes a line of Milton, a line of Pepys, a dash of Epictetus and some contemporary advertising:

> *The book you have in your hands,*
> *Confers the most benefits,*
> *By seeking to reduce regulatory burdens,*
> *The spirit of Plato to unfold.*
> *Full of rag-tag and bobtail,*
> *Dancing, singing and drinking,*
> *By which we are able to bear*
> *What comes to pass*
> *Without being crushed or depressed thereby;*
> *I used your product and have never looked back.*

Today I ask for understanding of the shortcomings of others and the ability to find the good in people and to appreciate their unique talents.

February 6th

On this day in 1564 the playwright Christopher Marlowe was born. Shakespeare was born the same year and the two are often compared. Marlowe's plays were hugely successful and he was, ostensibly, the better educated of the two since he went to Cambridge, whereas Shakespeare's formal education ended when he left school aged 18 and had to marry an already pregnant Anne Hathaway.

There is so little substantive evidence for the lives of both Marlowe and Shakespeare that we shall probably never get answers to many questions about their lives and deaths. What we do have for them though, is much of their written output. While Shakespeare normally comes out as top poet, Marlowe's work is extremely fine.

Here is Marlowe's Dr Faustus meeting Helen of Troy:

> Was this the face that launched a thousand ships
> And burnt the topless towers of Ilium?
> Sweet Helen, make me immortal with a kiss.
> Her lips suck forth my soul; see where it flies!
> Come, Helen, come, give me my soul again.
> Here will I dwell, for Heaven is in these lips,
> And all is dross that is not Helena.

And here is Shakespeare's Troilus meeting Cressida:

> I am giddy; expectation whirls me round.
> The imaginary relish is so sweet
> That it enchants my sense: what will it be,
> When that the watery palate tastes indeed
> Love's thrice ruptured nectar?

I think I prefer Marlowe in this instance.

Today I will try to be objective and not be hasty to judge others.

February 7th

On this day in 1478 Sir Thomas More, humanist, writer and statesman was born. More was a great scholar and a pious man who had, in his twenties, considered entering a monastery. His writings, especially Utopia, the imaginary land where laws were made on the basis of reason and a kind of communism was practised, brought him to the attention of King Henry VIII. More rose to become the king's chief advisor.

Later, however, Henry began his tortuous quest to find justification in the eyes of the church, for his divorce from his first wife, Catherine of Aragon. Eventually More had to choose between his King and his religious beliefs. He chose the latter and the consequences were dire. He was imprisoned, tried for treason and executed by a furious Henry. His final words were:

"The king's good servant, but God's first."

During his imprisonment he wrote some verses:

Eye-flattering Fortune! Look thou ne'er so fair,
Or ne'er so pleasantly begin to smile,
As though thou wouldst my ruin all repair,
During my life thou shalt not me beguile;
Trust shall I God to enter in erewhile,
His haven of havens sure and uniform:
After a calm I still expect the storm.
Long was I, Lady Luck, your serving-man,
And now have lost again all that I gat;
When, therefore, I think of you now and then,
And in my mind remember this and that,
Ye may not blame me, though I shrew your cat;
In faith I bless you, and a thousand times,
For lending me some leisure to make rhymes.

Today I will try to learn from the example of those who have difficult choices to make and manage to choose the right one.

February 8th

On this day in 1587 Mary Queen of Scots was beheaded at Fotheringhay Castle in Northamptonshire. When her time came she appeared serene and smiling but angrily refused the attentions of a Protestant cleric. When they lifted her body, her pet dog, a Skye terrier, was found hiding beneath her skirts.

Reactions to Mary's death were surprising, though probably politically motivated. Elizabeth, who had signed the death warrant, professed herself to be furious that she was not informed of the execution. In Scotland, Mary's son James, seeing himself in line for the English throne, is said to have barely reacted at all but to have 'continued with his hunting and other pastimes'. It could be said that Mary was lucky to have had a quick death. The conspirators in the Babington plot to kill Elizabeth (Mary's alleged involvement was the reason for her execution) were brutally eviscerated, hung, drawn and quartered at the Tower of London.

This poem, *The Housedove*, was written by conspirator Chidiock Tichbourne:

> *A silly housedove happed to fall*
> *Amongst a flock of crows,*
> *Which fed and filled her harmless craw*
> *Amongst her fatal foes.*
> *The crafty fowler drew his net –*
> *All his that he could catch –*
> *The crows lament their hellish chance,*
> *The dove repents her match.*
> *But too, too late! It was her chance*
> *The fowler did her spy,*
> *And so did take her for a crow –*
> *Which thing caused her to die.*

Today I ask that I will be steadfast and brave in all adversity and not seek to blame others.

February 9th

On this day in 1874 the American poet Amy Lowell was born. By all accounts Lowell was a short and rather plump lady. Ezra Pound is said to have unkindly called her the "hippopoetess".

A spinster, a feminist and apparently a lesbian, Lowell belied her patrician background by producing poetry full of pent up emotion and colourful imagery. TS Eliot called her "the demon saleswoman of poetry".

Here is part of her poem, *In Excelsis*:

You – you –
Your shadow is sunlight on a plate of silver;
Your footsteps, the seeding-place of lilies;
Your hands moving, a chime of bells across a windless air.
The movement of your hands is the long, golden running of
light from a rising sun;
It is the hopping of birds upon a garden-path.
As the perfume of jonquils, you come forth in the morning.
Young horses are not more sudden than your thoughts,
Your words are bees about a pear-tree,
Your fancies are the gold-and-black striped wasps buzzing
among red apples.
I drink your lips,
I eat the whiteness of your hands and feet.
My mouth is open. As a new jar I am empty and open.
How has the rainbow fallen upon my heart?
How have I snared the seas to lie in my fingers
And caught the sky to be a cover for my head? How have you
come to dwell with me,
Compassing me with the four circles of your mystic lightness,
So that I say "Glory! Glory!" and bow before you as to a
shrine?

Today I am grateful to live in a world where passion can be expressed.

February 10th

O n this day in 1609 the Cavalier poet Sir John Suckling was born. A soldier as well as a poet, he is famous as the inventor of the card game cribbage. He is said to have hit upon the plan of sending packs of marked playing cards to several of the stately homes in the land and then travelling around the country playing cribbage and amassing a huge fortune.

Suckling's short life had many ups and downs but after falling on hard times, he is believed to have poisoned himself in Paris, aged 32, rather than face living in poverty.

His opportunist attitude appears in his poetry:
Why so pale and wan, fond lover?
  Prithee, why so pale?
Will, when looking well can't move her,
  Looking ill prevail?
  Prithee, why so pale?
Why so dull and mute, young sinner?
  Prithee, why so mute?
Will, when speaking well can't win her,
  Saying nothing do 't?
  Prithee, why so mute?
Quit, quit for shame! This will not move;
  This cannot take her.
If of herself she will not love,
  Nothing can make her:
  The devil take her!

Today I will remember the distinction between pleasure and happiness and not pursue the first at the expense of the second.

February 11th

O n this day in 1858 Bernadette Soubirous, aged 14, saw the first of a series of visions at Lourdes. Bernadette, her sister and a friend were looking for firewood outside the town. She saw a small lady in a cave, dressed in blue and white. She never said she saw the Virgin Mary but constantly referred to 'Aquero', the patois word for 'that'.

Bernadette's visions were soon being witnessed by thousands and the Catholic Church, though at first sceptical, became convinced that something miraculous was happening at Lourdes. As indeed it was. Today five million people each year come to the little town which has more hotels than anywhere in France except Paris.

In 1933 Bernadette was declared a saint. Here are some things she said. They make a kind of poem:

> *Nothing very much.*
> *I don't think I've cured anyone whatsoever, and besides I*
> *haven't done anything for that reason.*
> *Oh, no, no. I want to stay poor.*
> *I heard a sound like a gust of wind.*
> *Then I turned my head towards the meadow.*
> *I saw the trees quite still: I went on taking off my stockings.*
> *I heard the same sound again.*
> *As I raised my head to look at the grotto,*
> *I saw a Lady dressed in white, wearing a white dress.*
> *I threw some holy water at her.*
> *They think I'm a saint . . . when I'm dead, they'll come and*
> *touch holy pictures and rosaries to me, and all the while I'll*
> *be getting broiled on a grill in purgatory.*
> *At least promise me you'll pray a lot for the repose of my*
> *soul.*

Today I am grateful for Bernadette whose example of humility, honesty, piety and love has inspired so many people who can see how much can be achieved with just these simple things.

February 12th

O n this day in 1809 the future US President Abraham Lincoln was born. From truly humble beginnings (born in a log cabin) Lincoln rose to become one of the world's most famous men. He presided through the civil war, arguably the most difficult period in the history of the United States and brought his country to peace and, to a great extent, forgiveness. He was also a charismatic leader and a gifted orator.

John Kennedy famously said of Churchill "he mobilised the English language and sent it into battle". He could have said the same of Lincoln. John Wilkes Booth, a disgruntled Confederate and actor who longed for immortality, is said to have killed Lincoln.

This poem, *The Glories of Our Blood and State*, by James Shirley says that only the actions of the just live on:

> *The glories of our blood and state*
> *Are shadows, not substantial things;*
> *There is no armour against Fate;*
> *Death lays his icy hand on kings:*
> *Sceptre and Crown*
> *Must tumble down,*
> *And in the dust be equal made*
> *With the poor crooked scythe and spade.*
> *The garlands wither on your brow;*
> *Then boast no more your mighty deeds!*
> *Upon Death's purple altar now*
> *See where the victor-victim bleeds.*
> *Your heads must come*
> *To the cold tomb:*
> *Only the actions of the just*
> *Smell sweet and blossom in their dust.*

Today I ask that the world be free of those prepared to use violence for their own ends.

February 13th

On this day in 1903 the Belgian writer Georges Simenon was born. Simenon will always be remembered for his creation, Commissaire Maigret, the cerebral and health conscious crime solver who was also an innately decent man. Whether the same could be same for his creator is another matter.

During the war he was suspected of being a German collaborateur and was later convicted for this. In his private life he had several mistresses and visited countless prostitutes. None of his marriages seems to have worked too well. Although Belgian by birth, Simenon spent most of his life in France and also lived in the USA for ten years after World War II.

Today's poem, *Conversation*, is by Frenchman Charles Baudelaire:

> You are a lovely, rosy, lucid autumn sky!
> But sadness mounts upon me like a flooding sea,
> And ebbs, and ebbing, leaves my lips morose and dry,
> Smarting with salty ooze, bitter with memory.
>
> – Useless to slide your hand like that along my breast;
> That which it seeks, my dear, is plundered; it is slit
> By the soft paw of woman, that clawed while it caressed.
> Useless to hunt my heart; the beasts have eaten it.
>
> My heart is like a palace where the mob has spat;
> There they carouse, they seize each other's hair, they kill.
> – Your breast is naked . . . what exotic scent is that?
>
> O Beauty, iron flail of souls, it is your will!
> So be it! Eyes of fire, bright in the darkness there,
> Bum up these strips of flesh the beasts saw fit to spare.

Today I will try my best to behave like an innately decent man.

February 14th

On this day the feast of St. Valentine is held. In early tradition, Valentine's Day was the date that birds began to choose their mates, only later did the romance extend to the human population.

The first reference in print to Valentine's Day is found in Geoffrey Chaucer's *The Parlement of Foules* (*The Parliament of Fowls*), in about 1381: "For this was on seynt Volantynys day Whan euery bryd comyth there to chese his mate." Nobody really knows who Saint Valentine was and why the date of 14th February was selected. It may relate to the engagement of King Richard II of England to Anne of Bohemia, which Chaucer's poem was written to honour.

The earliest known romantic Valentine verse was written by Charles, Duke of Orleans to his wife, in the 15th century:

> *Je suis desja d'amour tanné*
> *Ma tres doulce Valentinée*
> *(I am already sick of love,*
> *My very gentle Valentine)*
>
> *In Hamlet, Shakespeare had Ophelia sing this risqué*
> *Valentine's Day verse:*
> *To-morrow is Saint Valentine's Day*
> *All in the morning betime,*
> *And I a maid at your window*
> *To be your Valentine.*
> *Then up he rose, and donned his clothes,*
> *And dupped the chamber door.*
> *Let in the maid that out a maid*
> *Never departed more.*

Today I will remember the words of St Paul: "Three things will last forever – faith, hope and love – and the greatest of these is love".

February 15th

On this day in 1564 the Italian astronomer and mathematician Galileo Galilei was born. Galileo has been called the Father of Modern Science although during his lifetime his main view on a heliocentric universe was disallowed by the powerful Roman Catholic Church, which stuck to the literal biblical interpretation of the earth as the centre of the universe. Galileo was only repeating the views of Copernicus from over one hundred years earlier, but nevertheless the inquisition in Rome decided that he must: "abstain completely from teaching or defending this doctrine and opinion or from discussing it." Furthermore, over a decade later, he was placed under house arrest for the rest of his life.

Here are some lines by the metaphysical poet John Donne who was well aware of the new science that Copernicus and Galileo were introducing:

> The new philosophy calls all in doubt,
> The element of fire is quite put out;
> The sun is lost and the earth, and no man's wit
> Can well direct him where to look for it.
> And freely men confess that this world's spent,
> When in the planets and the firmament
> They seek so many new; they see that this
> Is crumbled out again to his atomies.
> Have not all souls thought
> For many ages that our body is wrought
> Of air and fire and other elements?
> And now they think of new ingredients;
> And one soul thinks one, and another way
> Another thinks, and 'tis an even lay.

Today I remember that that there are still huge questions to which we have no answer and when I look at the stars I remind myself that I am just a very small part of a vast joined-up universe.

February 16th

On this day in 1923 the Egyptologist Howard Carter opened the inner burial chamber of the Pharaoh Tutankhamen's tomb – this was the first Pharaoh's tomb to be found un-desecrated. There were many wonders within the tomb including a beautiful cup with the inscription "May your spirit live, May you spend millions of years, You who love Thebes, Sitting with your face to the north wind, Your eyes beholding happiness".

It was a historic moment but the joy was short lived. Many of those who were there that day met unexpected deaths soon after, including Lord Carnarvon who died two months later, of an infected mosquito bite. The very same day, his pet canary was killed by a cobra and back home in England his dog died.

Howard Carter lived on unscathed and died a natural death at the age of 64. It seemed that King Tut had spared him. In the prosaic setting of Putney Vale Cemetery in London, his gravestone is inscribed with familiar words: "May your spirit live, May you spend millions of years, You who love Thebes, Sitting with your face to the north wind, Your eyes beholding happiness."

Today's poem is from the Egyptian *Book of the Dead* written in 3500 BC, *He Biddeth Osiris to Arise from the Dead*:

> *Arise up on thy feet, O quiet heart.*
> *O Quiet Heart, thy body is made perfect.*
> *Isis among the reeds along the Nile*
> *And in the dark papyrus swamps bewailed thee,*
> *And sheltered Horus to avenge thy fate.*
> *He hath come forth from secret habitations,*
> *He hath warred mightily against thy foe,*
> *And now he saileth in the boat of sunrise.*
> *Come forth, O Quiet Heart, I have avenged thee.*

Today I will remember thanks for the lessons of history.

February 17th

On this day in 1864 the Australian poet, lawyer and journalist Andrew Barton (Banjo) Paterson was born. He is best known for writing what has now become the national song *Waltzing Matilda*. Brought up on a bush farm in New South Wales, Paterson attended Sydney Grammar School and then practised law before serving as an ambulance driver in France during World War I.

He was fond of horse racing too; here is part of his famous ballad *Old Pardon, the Son of Reprieve*:

> *You never heard tell of the story?*
> *Well, now, I can hardly believe!*
> *Never heard of the honour and glory*
> *Of Pardon, the son of Reprieve?*
> *But maybe you're only a Johnnie*
> *And don't know a horse from a hoe?*
> *Well, well, don't get angry, my sonny,*
> *But, really, a young un should know.*
> *They bred him out back on the 'Never',*
> *His mother was Mameluke breed.*
> *To the front – and then stay there – was ever*
> *The root of the Mameluke creed.*
> *He seemed to inherit their wiry*
> *Strong frames – and their pluck to receive –*
> *As hard as a flint and as fiery*
> *Was Pardon, the son of Reprieve.*
> *We ran him at many a meeting*
> *At crossing and gully and town,*
> *And nothing could give him a beating –*
> *At least when our money was down . . .*

Today I will try to make this a good day knowing that I can offer a positive attitude when I make this happen.

February 18th

On this day in 1564 Michelangelo Buonarroti died aged 88. He spent years painting the ceiling of the Sistine Chapel, in the Vatican. The project was physically and emotionally devastating. Michelangelo recounts its effect on him with these words: "After four tortured years, more than 400 over life-sized figures, I felt as old and as weary as Jeremiah. I was only 37, yet friends did not recognise the old man I had become."

Perhaps equally remarkable was that he didn't much like painting anyway, considering sculpture to be an infinitely superior art. One of the qualities most admired by his contemporaries was his "terribilità", a sense of awe-inspiring grandeur. Anyone who has seen his sculpture 'David' will understand why. During their lifetimes Michelangelo and Leonardo da Vinci were rivals.

Opinions are still divided on who was superior, though Leonardo took himself off to France for the last years of his life on a series of commissions which put an end to the rivalry. Perhaps he suspected that he might not win the vote. It is however fruitless to sit in judgement on two such great artists and we should just be grateful for them both.

Here is a poem, *Heraclitus* by William Cory, about loss, that I think is justly admired for its underlying feeling of regret and nostalgia:

> They told me, Heraclitus, they told me you were dead,
> They brought me bitter news to hear and bitter tears to shed.
> I wept, as I remembered, how often you and I
> Had tired the sun with talking and sent him down the sky.
> And now that thou art lying, my dear old Carian guest,
> A handful of grey ashes, long ago at rest,
> Still are thy pleasant voices, thy nightingales, awake;
> For Death, he taketh all away, but them he cannot take.

Today I give thanks for all the man-made beauty in the world and for the people who worked to produce it.

February 19th

On this day in 1949 American expatriate Ezra Pound won the Bollingen Prize for poetry. Pound was a major figure in literary circles between the wars and helped many struggling writers to achieve recognition including Eliot, Hemingway and Joyce. Before World War II Pound lost trust in democracy and in Italy during the war he became an advocate of Fascism, which caused him to be imprisoned and ill-treated after the war ended.

His own poetry is difficult to judge. It is intellectual and shows his vast scholarship and range of interests with often intense imagery. It can however, be difficult to fathom – perhaps that was his intention. Certainly many people think that Pound did more for modern poetry in the English language than anyone else.

Here is a poem by James Weldon Johnson, a poet with a modern style, *Deep In the Quiet Wood*:

> *Are you bowed down in heart?*
> *Do you but hear the clashing discords and the din of life?*
> *Then come away, come to the peaceful wood,*
> *Here bathe your soul in silence. Listen! Now,*
> *From out the palpitating solitude*
> *Do you not catch, yet faint, elusive strains?*
> *They are above, around, within you, everywhere.*
> *Silently listen! Clear, and still more clear, they come.*
> *They bubble up in rippling notes, and swell in singing tones.*
> *Not let your soul run the whole gamut of the wondrous scale*
> *Until, responsive to the tonic chord,*
> *It touches the diapason of God's grand cathedral organ,*
> *Filling earth for you with heavenly peace*
> *And holy harmonies.*

Today I ask to learn new and deeper meanings to life and I will continue to read poetry with an enquiring mind.

February 20th

On this day in 1950 the Welsh poet Dylan Thomas arrived in New York City for the start of his first poetry reading tour. There were four tours in all which provided a valuable income for the family, who were chronically poor. The downside was that it gave Dylan freedom to drink and philander, away from the watchful eye of his wife, Caitlin (though her own behaviour when alone often mirrored his).

The fourth tour was disastrous from the start, with Thomas almost permanently drunk and suffering from gout and blackouts. He collapsed at the Chelsea Hotel and was admitted to hospital in a coma with 'acute alcoholic encephalopathy'. Caitlin flew over and, after a drunken rage at the hospital, was put in a straitjacket and sent to an alcohol detox unit. Dylan Thomas never recovered consciousness and died the next day. Caitlin went on to marry again and died in Italy, aged 80. She had been attending Alcoholics Anonymous for over 20 years.

This poem, *Chain of Pearls by Rabindranath Tagore*, has for me a slight flavour of some of Thomas's work:

> *Mother, I shall weave a chain of pearls for thy neck*
> *With my tears of sorrow.*
> *The stars have wrought their anklets of light to deck thy feet,*
> *But mine will hang upon thy breast.*
> *Wealth and fame come from thee*
> *And it is for thee to give or to withhold them.*
> *But this my sorrow is absolutely mine own,*
> *And when I bring it to thee as my offering*
> *Thou rewardest me with thy grace.*

Today I recognise the hell of addiction and give thanks that I no longer need to take mood altering substances.

February 21st

On this day in 1925 the first issue of the *New Yorker* magazine appeared. All articles are to a very high standard and facts are carefully checked (it employed 16 fact checkers). Most of the great names have contributed over the years – Salinger, Fitzgerald, Updike, Thurber, and Murakami are a few. It has not shrunk from controversy; the biggest ever response from readers was to the 1949 story *The Lottery*, a sinister tale of a fictional Midwest village where an annual rite of a 'lottery' chose the person to be stoned to death, so as to ensure a good harvest.

Of the thousands who wrote in, many seemed to want to know where they could watch the event. It is also famous for its cartoons.

Here is a poem by Alfred Lord Tennyson, whose work was featured in the *New Yorker* in 1939, with illustrations by cartoonist James Thurber, Summer Night:

> *Now sleeps the crimson petal, now the white;*
> *Nor waves the cypress in the palace walk;*
> *Nor winks the gold fin in the porphyry font:*
> *The firefly wakens: waken thou with me.*
> *　　Now droops the milk-white peacock like a ghost,*
> *And like a ghost she glimmers on to me.*
> *　　Now lies the Earth all Danae to the stars,*
> *And all thy heart lies open unto me.*
> *　　Now slides the silent meteor on, and leaves*
> *A shining furrow, as thy thoughts in me.*
> *　　Now folds the lily all her sweetness up,*
> *And slips into the bosom of the lake:*
> *So fold thyself, my dearest, thou, and slip*
> *Into my bosom and be lost in me.*

Today I give thanks for the beauty of poetry and those who bring it to our attention.

February 22nd

On this day in 1892 the American lyrical poet Edna St. Vincent Millay was born. Raised in Rural Maine, Millay moved to New York City after graduating from Vassar.
Openly bisexual, she lived for some years a life of parties and pleasure.

Her poetry is about love and relationships and often has a sad tone combined with powerful imagery. Here is one:

> And do you think that love itself,
> Living in such an ugly house,
> Can prosper long?
> We meet and part;
> Our talk is all of heres and nows,
> Our conduct likewise; in no act
> Is any future, any past;
> Under our sly, unspoken pact,
> I know with whom I saw you last,
> But I say nothing; and you know
> At six-fifteen to whom I go –
> Can even love be treated so?
> I know but I do not insist,
> Having stealth and tact, thought not enough,
> What hour your eye is on your wrist.
> No wild appeal, no mild rebuff
> Deflates the hour, leaves the wine flat –
> Yet if you drop the picked-up book
> To intercept my clockward look –
> Tell me, can love go on like that?
> Even the bored, insulted heart,
> That signed so long and tight a lease,
> Can break its contract slump in peace.

Today I will try to appreciate the little things in life.

February 23rd

On this day in 1633 the English diarist Samuel Pepys was born. Sometimes he comforted himself at night as when he dreamt, during the terrible year of the great plague, that he was with the King's favourite mistress, Lady Castlemaine: "The best that ever was dreamed – which was, that I had my Lady Castlemayne in my arms and was admitted to use all the dalliance I desired with her, and then dreamed that this could not be awake but that it was only a dream. But that since it was a dream and that I took so much real pleasure in it, what a happy thing it would be, if when we are in our graves (as Shakespeare resembles it), we could dream, and dream but such dreams as this – that then we should not need to be so fearful of death as we are this plague-time."

Today's poem is by John Donne, who lived through plagues before Pepys was born:

> Go and catch a falling star,
> Get with child a mandrake root,
> Tell me where all past years are,
> Or who cleft the devil's foot,
> Teach me to hear mermaids singing,
> Or to keep off envy's stinging,
> And find, what wind
> Serves to advance an honest mind.
> If thou be'st born to strange sights,
> Things invisible to see,
> Ride ten thousand days and nights,
> Till age snow white hairs on thee,
> Thou, when thou return'st, wilt tell me,
> All strange wonders that befell thee,
> And swear, no where
> Lives a woman true and fair.

Today I ask that I will never lose my enjoyment and appreciation of life, even in the face of disaster.

February 24th

On this day in 1809 the Drury Lane Theatre, owned by the playwright Richard Brinsley Sheridan, was burnt down. Sheridan sat in an armchair with a glass of wine to watch it burn saying: "A man may surely be allowed to take a glass of wine by his own fireside."

Known for his ready wit, he wrote several delightful plays that are still regularly performed today. Most popular are *The Rivals* and *The School for Scandal*. The fire ruined Sheridan financially and he died with many debts although he knew most of the leading figures of the time, such as the Prince of Wales and Dr Samuel Johnson and was popular in society. He is buried at Westminster Abbey in Poets' Corner.

Here is one of his poems:

Had I a heart for falsehood framed,
I ne'er could injure you;
For though your tongue no promise claimed,
Your charms would make me true:
To you no soul shall bear deceit,
No stranger offer wrong;
But friends in all the aged you'll meet,
And lovers in the young.
For when they learn that you have blest
Another with your heart,
They'll bid aspiring passion rest,
And act a brother's part;
Then, lady, dread not here deceit,
Nor fear to suffer wrong;
For friends in all the aged you'll meet,
And lovers in the young.

Today I give thanks for my family and friends and for all the wit and the happiness that they bring.

February 25th

On this day in 1841 the French artist Pierre Auguste Renoir was born in Limoges. As a youth, he worked in the famous local porcelain factory as a designer before moving to Paris aged 21 to study art. Initially he struggled for success, like so many of his fellow artists and friends such as Monet, Sisley and Pissarro who joined together in the Impressionist movement.

However, after exhibiting at the first Impressionist exhibition in 1874, Renoir gained recognition and soon became a fashionable painter. During his life he produced thousands of works and continued painting almost until his death aged 78 – despite being so crippled by rheumatoid arthritis that assistants would have to place the brush into his hand.

Renoir was influenced by the work of Delacroix, Courbet and Boucher and shortly before his death visited the Louvre to see his paintings hanging alongside the old masters. Great art of any kind can inspire great poetry. Here is John Keats's sonnet *On First Looking into Chapman's Homer*:

> *Much have I travell'd in the realms of gold,*
>   *And many goodly states and kingdoms seen;*
>   *Round many western islands have I been*
> *Which bards in fealty to Apollo hold.*
> *Oft of one wide expanse had I been told*
>   *That deep-brow'd Homer ruled as his demesne;*
>   *Yet did I never breathe its pure serene*
> *Till I heard Chapman speak out loud and bold:*
> *Then felt I like some watcher of the skies*
>   *When a new planet swims into his ken;*
> *Or like stout Cortez when with eagle eyes*
>   *He star'd at the Pacific—and all his men*
> *Look'd at each other with a wild surmise—*
>   *Silent, upon a peak in Darien.*

Today I am grateful for the beauty that is brought into the world through art of all kinds.

February 26th

On this day in 1802 the French novelist Victor Marie Hugo was born. His father was an officer in the French army. These were interesting times – Napoleon had been in power for two years when he was born and the Battle of Waterloo took place when he was 13.

Young Victor saw many places due to his father's postings with the army. After he married, the family was beset by tragedy, when his daughter was drowned in a boating accident aged 20.

A devastated Victor wrote several heart rending poems – here is one, *Demain, dès l'aube*:

> *Tomorrow, at dawn, the moment daylight touches the land,*
> *I will leave. You see, I know that you wait for me.*
> *I will go through forest, I will go across the mountains.*
> *I cannot rest far from you for long.*
> *I will trudge on, my eyes fixed on my thoughts,*
> *Without seeing outside of myself, without hearing any sound,*
> *Alone, unknown, back bent, hands crossed,*
> *Sad, and the day for me will be like the night.*
> *I will not look upon the golden sunset as night falls,*
> *Nor the sailboats from afar that descend on Harfleur,*
> *And when I arrive, I will place on your grave*
> *A bouquet of green holly and heather in bloom.*

Victor Hugo became a national treasure during his lifetime and the Avenue d'Eylau where he lived was renamed Avenue Victor Hugo. Letters to him were thenceforth addressed: 'To M. Victor Hugo, In his Avenue, Paris'. It would be a poor French town today that does not have a street bearing his name. When he died, two million people joined his funeral procession from the Arc de Triomphe to the Pantheon.

Today I reflect on the ability to love: to recognise the feeling and be able to show it.

February 27th

On this day in 1807 the American poet Henry Wadsworth Longfellow was born. An academic and for a time a professor at Harvard, he is known for his ballads *The Song of Hiawatha* and *Paul Revere's Ride*.

Longfellow's life sometimes appears superficial compared to the angst and torment endured by some poets, but he did endure some emotional pain, especially over the untimely death in 1861 of Frances who was badly burnt and died following an accident with matches (not unusual at a time of open fires, candles and long dresses).

Here is his only love poem, to his second wife, Frances Appleton:

> Lo! In the painted oriel of the West,
>   Whose panes the sunken sun incarnadines,
>   Like a fair lady at her casement, shines
>   The evening star, the star of love and rest!
> And then anon she doth herself divest
>   Of all her radiant garments, and reclines
>   Behind the sombre screen of yonder pines,
>   With slumber and soft dreams of love oppressed.
> O my beloved, my sweet Hesperus!
>   My morning and my evening star of love!
>   My best and gentlest lady! Even thus,
> As that fair planet in the sky above,
>   Dost thou retire unto thy rest at night,
>   And from thy darkened window fades the light.

Today I ask to understand the meaning of true love and friendship.

February 28th

On this day in 2002 the currencies of 11 participating European countries were cancelled as legal tender marking the official start of the Euro as the sole Eurozone currency. Nothing on such a scale had been attempted before. Many of the smaller member countries felt an immediate benefit. Whether the Euro remains a success story or indeed remains at all is still an open question. Britain remains the most notable European outsider and a succession of Prime Ministers have endured criticism from their European counterparts for their steadfastly insular refusal to join the party.

In retrospect, they seem to have acted wisely and Sterling remains a strong and manageable currency worldwide.

Today's poem by Dante Gabriel Rossetti is suitably titled *On a Handful of French Money*:

> These coins that jostle on my hand do own
> No single image: each name here and date
> Denoting in man's consciousness and state
> New change. In some, the face is clearly known, –
> In others marred. The badge of that old throne
> Of Kings is on the obverse; or this sign
> Which says, "I France am all – lo, I am mine!"
> Or else the Eagle that dared soar alone.
> Even as these coins, so are these lives and years
> Mixed and bewildered; yet hath each of them
> No less its part in what is come to be
> For France. Empire, Republic, Monarchy, –
> Each clamours or keeps silence in her name,
> And lives within the pulse that now is hers.

Today I reflect on the meaning of money and its true value and benefit to mankind, if any. Would we be happier without it?

February 29th

O n this day in 1789 the composer and pianist Frederic Chopin was born in Warsaw. Chopin's name is much linked with George Sand, the diminutive but feisty cross-dressing authoress. Chopin would often spend summers at Sand's country estate at Nohan, in France, where life was relaxed. The painter Delacroix was another visitor: "The hosts could not be more pleasant in entertaining me. When we are not all together at dinner, lunch, playing billiards, or walking, each of us stays in his room, reading or lounging around on a couch. Sometimes, through the window which opens on the garden, a gust of music wafts up from Chopin at work. All this mingles with the songs of nightingales and the fragrance of roses."

Sadly, Chopin and Sand quarrelled and their relationship ended. Chopin's work and output is said to have suffered. How much Sand was an inspiration to him we do not know.

Here is a rather strange poem to Chopin by Emma Lazarus:

> *A dream of interlinking hands, of feet*
> *Tireless to spin the unseen, fairy woof*
> *Of the entangling waltz. Bright eyebeams meet,*
> *Gay laughter echoes from the vaulted roof.*
> *Warm perfumes rise; the soft unflickering glow*
> *Of branching lights sets off the changeful charms*
> *Of glancing gems, rich stuffs, the dazzling snow*
> *Of necks unkerchieft, and bare, clinging arms.*
> *Hark to the music! How beneath the strain*
> *Of reckless revelry, vibrates and sobs*
> *One fundamental chord of constant pain,*
> *The pulse-beat of the poet's heart that throbs.*
> *So yearns, though all the dancing waves rejoice,*
> *The troubled sea's disconsolate, deep voice.*

Today I will remember that serenity, courage and wisdom are all that I need to cope with life.

March 1st

On this day in 1445, the first day of Spring, the Florentine painter Alessandro Botticelli was born. Much of his work was done for his patrons, the Medici family, though he also produced work for the Pope's Sistine Chapel in Rome. Botticelli produced some amazingly lyrical allegorical works such as *The Birth of Venus* and *Primavera* (Spring) and some delightful portraits.

Later, like many in Florence at the time, he came under the influence of the stern and moralistic friar Savonarola and may have burnt some of his works because they were on pagan themes. Botticelli is said to have harboured an unrequited love for Simonetta Vespucci, the model for 'Venus', a beautiful married lady who died at the age of 22. He requested to be buried at her feet when he died and this was carried out.

Today's poem is on the subject of Spring, by Gerard Manley Hopkins:

Nothing is so beautiful as spring –
  When weeds, in wheels, shoot long and lovely and lush;
  Thrush's eggs look little low heavens, and thrush
Through the echoing timber does so rinse and wring
The ear, it strikes like lightnings to hear him sing;
  The glassy peartree leaves and blooms, they brush
  The descending blue; that blue is all in a rush
With richness; the racing lambs too have fair their fling.
What is all this juice and all this joy?
  A strain of the earth's sweet being in the beginning
In Eden garden. – Have, get, before it cloy,
  Before it cloud, Christ, lord, and sour with sinning,
Innocent mind and Mayday in girl and boy,
  Most, O maid's child, thy choice and worthy the winning.

Today I reflect on springtime and the renewal of life that it signifies.

March 2nd

On this day in 1931 the writer and journalist Tom Wolfe was born. Wolfe excelled both academically and at baseball – he considered turning professional. He favoured saturation reporting where the journalist spends huge amounts of time involved in a subject's life.

His masterpiece is probably the novel Bonfire of the Vanities, which he wrote as weekly instalments in Rolling Stone magazine, deliberately copying the method that Dickens and Thackeray had pioneered a century earlier. The book was a huge success. Its title comes from the famous 1497 Bonfire of the Vanities that took place in Florence.

This poem, a small part of it, by modernist poet Don Marquis, *Unrest*, would have resonated with Wolfe:

> *A fierce unrest seethes at the core*
> *Of all existing things:*
> *It was the eager wish to soar*
> *That gave the gods their wings.*
> *From what flat wastes of cosmic slime,*
> *And stung by what quick fire,*
> *Sunward the restless races climb! –*
> *Men risen out of mire!*
> *There throbs through all the worlds that are*
> *This heart-beat hot and strong,*
> *And shaken systems, star by star,*
> *Awake and glow in song.*
> *But for the urge of this unrest*
> *These joyous spheres are mute;*
> *But for the rebel in his breast*
> *Had man remained a brute.*

Today I will practise mindfulness as a way of living one day at a time, because the past cannot be changed and the future may never happen.

March 3rd

On this day in 1847 the inventor Alexander Graham Bell was born. Although credited with inventing the telephone, Bell always considered it an intrusion on his real work as a scientist and refused to have one in his study.

He had been interested in 'inventing' since his childhood in Edinburgh. Much of his early work was helping deaf people and he wrote books on sign language and lip reading.

This is part of a poem which describes how news was delivered before Bell's time. It has a rousing rhythm and it is a quite a harrowing story, especially for the horses: *How We Brought the Good News from Ghent to Aix*, by Robert Browning:

> I sprang to the stirrup, and Joris, and he;
>   I galloped, Dirck galloped, we galloped all three;
>   "Good speed!" cried the watch as the gate-bolts undrew;
>   "Speed!" echoed the wall to us galloping through;
>   Behind shut the postern, the lights sank to rest,
>   And into the midnight we galloped abreast.
>   Not a word to each other; we kept the great pace
>   Neck by neck, stride by stride, never changing our place;
>   I turned in my saddle and made its girth tight,
>   Then shortened each stirrup, and set the pique right,
>   Rebuckled the cheek-strap, chained slacker the bit,
>   Nor galloped less steadily Roland a whit.
>   So Joris broke silence with, "Yet there is time!"
>   By Hasselt, Dirck groaned; and cried Joris, "Stay spur!
>   Your Roos galloped bravely, the fault's not in her,
>   We'll remember at Aix" – for one heard the quick wheeze
>   Of her chest, saw the stretched neck and staggering knees,
>   And sunk tail, and horrible heave of the flank,
>   As down on her haunches she shuddered and sank.

Today I will focus on being able to communicate in a simple and direct way in the interests of mutual understanding.

March 4th

On this day in 1963 the poet William Carlos Williams died. Williams lived in New Jersey and was also a doctor, practicing medicine by day and writing poems at night. He began publishing modernist poetry in his 20s but considered himself upstaged by the poet TS Eliot, who was also a friend and whose poetry was appearing at this time.

Williams's own poetry focused on basic American words and idioms and aimed at producing a new 'transatlantic' form of poetry which dealt with every day occurrences in the lives of ordinary people.

Here is part of a poem by JK Stephen who lived in England and whose work has some of the wit of Williams:

> *I am not ambitious at all:*
> *I am not a poet, I know*
> *(Though I do love to see a mere scrawl*
> *To order and symmetry grow).*
> *My muse is uncertain and slow,*
> *I am not expert with my tools,*
> *I lack the poetic argot:*
> *But I hope I have kept to the rules.*
> *When your brain is undoubtedly small,*
> *'Tis hard, sir, to write in a row,*
> *Some five or six rhymes to Nepaul,*
> *And more than a dozen to Joe:*
> *The metre is easier though,*
> *Three rhymes are sufficient for 'ghouls,'*
> *My lines are deficient in go,*
> *But I hope I have kept to the rules. Dear Sir, though my*
> *language is low,*
> *Let me dip in Pierian pools:*
> *My verses are only so so,*
> *But I hope I have kept to the rules.*

Today I will try not to allow my feelings to dictate my actions.

March 5th

On this day in 1894 Archibald Philip Primrose, 5th Earl of Rosebery, became Prime Minister of Britain. It was said that he was too patrician to handle the democratic process or, as Winston Churchill quipped at the time: 'he would not stoop, he did not conquer.'

Rosebery was born to a life of privilege and chose to leave university early rather than give up the racehorse that he had purchased (not allowed, even at Oxford). He married Hannah Rothschild, said to be the richest woman in England, and was devastated when she died. A keen sports lover, he won the Epsom Derby three times and supported Scotland's football team to such an extent that they sometimes turned out wearing his racing colours of primrose and pink.

Rosebery achieved his three stated childhood ambitions: to win the Derby, marry an heiress and be Prime Minister. He died at home aged 82 listening to a recording of the Eton Boating Song – his last request.

Here is part of it, composed by Eton master William Johnson in 1862:

> Jolly boating weather,
> And a hay harvest breeze,
> Blade on the feather,
> Shade off the trees,
>   Swing swing together,
>   With your bodies between your knees. Twenty years hence
> this weather,
> May tempt us from office stools,
> We may be slow on the feather,
> And seem to the boys old fools,
>   But we'll still swing together,
>   And swear by the best of schools.

Today I will be grateful for all the gifts that I have been given.

March 6th

On this day in 1927 the Colombian writer Gabriel Garcia Marquez was born. Known as Gabo for short by his millions of admirers, he wrote several of South America's defining novels including *Love in the Time of Cholera* and *One Hundred Years of Solitude*, the latter being Marquez's first major novel.

To write it he had to sell his car and put his family into debt for a year, but happily the book was and still is considered a masterpiece. It won him the Nobel Prize for literature. His style has been described as 'magic realism', whereby an element of magic is brought into mundane and otherwise realistic events.

This poem, *In Time of Plague* by Thomas Nashe has some of the flavour of Marquez:

Adieu, farewell, earth's bliss;
This world uncertain is;
Fond are life's lustful joys;
Death proves them all but toys;
None from his darts can fly;
I am sick, I must die.
  Lord, have mercy on us!
Rich men, trust not in wealth,
Gold cannot buy you health;
Physic himself must fade.
All things to end are made,
The plague full swift goes by;
I am sick, I must die.

  Lord, have mercy on us!
Beauty is but a flower
Which wrinkles will devour;
Brightness falls from the air;
Queens have died young and fair;
Dust hath closed Helen's eye.
I am sick, I must die.
  Lord, have mercy on us!
Haste, therefore, each degree,
To welcome destiny;
Heaven is our heritage,
Earth but a player's stage;
Mount we unto the sky.
I am sick, I must die.
  Lord, have mercy on us.

Today I will try to bring an element of magic realism into my own life, and into the lives of others.

March 7th

On this day in 1872 the Dutch painter Piet Mondrian was born. Though he started by painting landscapes, Mondrian was greatly influenced by the work of the cubists, especially Picasso and Braque, and saw abstraction as a way for art to transcend reality.

After attending art school he worked in The Netherlands before leaving in 1911 to live in Paris where his paintings became more geometric. He was also a member of the Theosophy movement and saw his work as seeking a deeper spiritual meaning to life.

Following the rise of Hitler, Mondrian moved to London and then to New York where he spent the last six years of his life. He died in 1944. Much of his work appears modern today though painted nearly a hundred years ago.

Here is a poem, *Sonnet* by Alan Seeger, about a different kind of modernity:

Down the strait vistas where a city street
Fades in pale dust and vaporous distances,
Stained with far fumes the light grows less and less
And the sky reddens round the day's retreat.
Now out of orient chambers, cool and sweet,
Like Nature's pure lustration, Dusk comes down.
Now the lamps brighten and the quickening town
Rings with the trample of returning feet.
And Pleasure, risen from her own warm mould
Sunk all the drowsy and unloved daylight
In layers of odorous softness, Paphian girls
Cover with gauze, with satin, and with pearls,
Crown, and about her spangly vestments fold
The ermine of the empire of the Night.

Today I will try not to be distracted or upset by the trivia and annoyances of modern life, but rather to be grateful for the benefits that I have received.

March 8th

On this day in 1859 the author Kenneth Grahame was born. Known for *The Wind in the Willows*, Graham drew on his own childhood experiences of 'messing about in boats' on the Thames.

Although he started writing and publishing articles as a young man he did not publish *The Wind in the Willows* until 1908, at the age of 49. This was the year that he left the Bank of England, where he had worked for 29 years.

There is only one possible choice for today's poem. It is *Mr Toad*. Grahame is said to have modelled his famous character on the behaviour of his deeply troubled son, Alastair:

> *The world has held great Heroes,*
> *As history-books have showed;*
> *But never a name to go down to fame*
> *Compared with that of Toad!*
> *The clever men at Oxford*
> *Know all that there is to be knowed.*
> *But they none of them know one half as much*
> *As intelligent Mr Toad!*
> *The animals sat in the Ark and cried,*
> *Their tears in torrents flowed.*
> *Who was it said, 'There's land ahead'?*
> *Encouraging Mr Toad!*
> *The army all saluted*
> *As they marched along the road.*
> *Was it the King? Or Kitchener?*
> *No. It was Mr Toad.*
> *The Queen and her Ladies-in-waiting*
> *Sat at the window and sewed.*
> *She cried, 'Look! Who's that handsome man?'*
> *They answered, 'Mr Toad.'*

Today I will try to keep things simple: to give and to receive in a direct and simple manner without manipulation.

March 9th

O n this day in 1892 the author, poet and gardener Vita Sackville West was born. Married to the brilliant writer and politician Sir Harold Nicholson with whom she had two children, Vita is famous for the series of passionate affairs that she conducted with people of both sexes.

'She was Lady Chatterley and her lover rolled into one', as one commentator put it. They had an open marriage, but a very happy one that seems to have lasted well and they were devoted to each other.

She wrote tender, emotional poetry to several lovers, including Virginia Woolf, and would certainly have known and appreciated this fragment from the Greek poetess Sappho, writing on the Isle of Lesbos around 600 BC – *Come to Me Here from Crete*:

> *Come to me here from Crete,*
> *To this holy temple, where*
> *Your lovely apple grove stands,*
> *And your altars that flicker*
> *With incense.*
> *And below the apple branches, cold*
> *Clear water sounds, everything shadowed*
> *By roses, and sleep that falls from*
> *Bright shaking leaves.*
> *And a pasture for horses blossoms*
> *With the flowers of spring, and breezes*
> *Are flowing here like honey:*
> *Come to me here,*
> *Here, Cyprian, delicately taking*
> *Nectar in golden cups*
> *Mixed with a festive joy,*
> *And pour.*

Today I give thanks for all the eccentrics and individuals in the world who are not afraid to show themselves as they are.

March 10th

On this day in 1948 Zelda Fitzgerald died in a fire at a mental hospital. She is often seen as a mere sidekick to the talented but doomed Scott Fitzgerald but she wrote one novel herself, some of which Scott plagiarised. At first they were feted as a golden couple, then gossiped about and finally seen as an embarrassment.

It was a stormy relationship and Scott's alcoholism as well as her mental instability caused many problems. When he died in 1940, in Hollywood, aged 44, they had not met for over a year.

Zelda was buried next to Scott. On the headstone are these ending lines from *The Great Gatsby*, arguably Scott's finest book: "So we beat on, boats against the current, borne back ceaselessly into the past."

Here is one of Scott's poems, *On A Play Twice Seen*:

> *Here in the figured dark I watch once more;*
> *There with the curtain rolls a year away,*
> *A year of years – there was an idle day*
> *Of ours, when happy endings didn't bore*
> *Our unfermented souls, and rocks held ore:*
> *Your little face beside me, wide-eyed, gay,*
> *Smiled its own repertoire, while the poor play*
> *Reached me as a faint ripple reaches shore.*
> *Yawning and wondering an evening through*
> *I watch alone – and chattering's of course*
> *Spoil the one scene which somehow did have charms;*
> *You wept a bit, and I grew sad for you*
> *Right there, where Mr. X defends divorce*
> *And What's-Her-Name falls fainting in his arms.*

Today I will try to set realistic goals for myself and I will remember that perfectionism can be an excuse to do nothing.

March 11th

On this day in 1952 English writer Douglas Adams was born. His extraordinary imagination and inventiveness reached its apex in the radio series *The Hitch-hikers Guide to the Galaxy* which he said began when he was lying drunk on a Swiss mountainside one night with a guide book in his pocket. He was also a campaigner for saving threatened animal species and climbed Mount Kilimanjaro in a rhino outfit to raise money. He died suddenly in California of a heart attack in 2001, aged 49. Somehow I always think of Adams when I read *The Cloud* by Percy Bysshe Shelley. Here are the last two verses:

> *Sunbeam-proof, I hang like a roof,*
> *The mountains its columns be.*
> *The triumphal arch through which I march*
> *With hurricane, fire, and snow,*
> *When the Powers of the air are chained to my chair,*
> *Is the million-coloured bow;*
> *The sphere-fire above its soft colours wove,*
> *While the moist Earth was laughing below.*
> *I am the daughter of Earth and Water,*
> *And the nursling of the Sky;*
> *I pass through the pores of the ocean and shores;*
> *I change, but I cannot die.*
> *For after the rain when with never a stain*
> *The pavilion of Heaven is bare,*
> *And the winds and sunbeams with their convex gleams*
> *Build up the blue dome of air,*
> *I silently laugh at my own cenotaph,*
> *And out of the caverns of rain,*
> *Like a child from the womb, like a ghost from the tomb,*
> *I arise and unbuild it again.*

Today I will try to be a giver rather than a taker: I will practice giving kindness, consideration and compassion to others.

March 12th

On this day in 1912 the Canadian poet Irving Layton was born. He is known for his combative 'tell it like it is' style that contrasted with the ornate imagery of the previous century's writing. He was married five times and seems to have had a distinctly chauvinistic view of the opposite sex, which incurred the wrath of the feminist movement.

This shows in his poems which have names like *Women are Stupid*. Layton died in a nursing home aged 93, controversial to the end. All his wives had already left him.

This poem *In the Backs*, is by another possible misogynist who was, for a time, suspected of being Jack the Ripper – James K. Stephen, cousin of Virginia Woolf:

> As I was strolling lonely in the Backs,
> I met a woman whom I did not like.
> I did not like the way the woman walked:
> Loose-hipped, big-boned, disjointed, angular.
> If her anatomy comprised a waist,
> I did not notice it: she had a face
> With eyes and lips adjusted thereunto,
> But round her mouth no pleasing shadows stirred,
> Nor did her eyes invite a second glance.
> And so she stalked her dull unthinking way;
> Or, if she thought of anything, it was
> That such a one had got a second class,
> Or Mrs So-and-So a second child.
> I did not want to see that girl again:
> I did not like her: and I should not mind
> If she were done away with, killed, or ploughed.
> She did not seem to serve a useful end:
> And certainly she was not beautiful.

Today I will try to give every person that I meet the respect to which they are entitled, regardless of race, sex or creed.

March 13th

On this day in 1913 the Greek diplomat and poet Georgios Seferiades was born. Using the pen name George Seferis, he wrote many beautiful verses that show the influence of the ancient Greeks such as Homer and Euripides as well as modern poets such as Eliot and Pound.

A diplomat, he was ambassador to Britain in the late fifties and worked hard to achieve a solution to the fighting between Greeks and Turks in Cyprus, an island that he particularly loved. He won the Nobel Prize for literature in 1963.

This poem, *Song to Celia* by Ben Johnson, harks back to the works of the Roman poet Catullus with whom Seferiades would have been familiar:

> *Drink to me, only, with thine eyes,*
> *And I will pledge with mine;*
> *Or leave a kisse but in the cup,*
> *And Ile not look for wine.*
> *The thirst, that from the soule doth rise,*
> *Doth aske a drink divine:*
> *But might I of Jove's Nectar sup,*
> *I would not change for thine.*
> *I sent thee, late, a rosie wreath,*
> *Not so much honoring thee,*
> *As giving it a hope, that there*
> *It could not withered be.*
> *But thou thereon did'st onely breathe,*
> *And sent'st it back to mee:*
> *Since when it growes, and smells, I sweare,*
> *Not of it selfe, but thee.*

Today I ask that I will learn to share myself, my qualities and my failings, with my family and friends.

March 14th

On this day in 1887 Sylvia Beach, the American publisher and bookseller, was born. Sylvia grew up in Baltimore, Maryland but came to Paris in 1901 when her father, a Presbyterian minister, was appointed to the American church there.

Beach opened her famous bookshop Shakespeare and Co in the 6th Arrondissement in 1919 after meeting and falling in love with Adrienne Monnier who owned a bookshop called La Maison des Amis du Livre in rue de l'Odeon. The two were to remain together for the next 36 years. Soon Beach moved her shop opposite to Monnier's, in the same street.

Shakespeare and Co became famous for first publishing James Joyce's *Ulysses* in 1922 when no one else would, though Beach lost a lot of money by doing so. Only one thousand copies were printed. Subsequently, the bookshop became a magnet for writers and publishers, particularly expatriates such as Hemingway, Eliot, Pound, DH Lawrence, and Man Ray. Although doing good business before World War II, it was forced to close when Paris fell to the Nazis and Beach was interned. She will always be honoured for the help that she gave to aspiring writers.

Here is a well-known poem, *There is no Frigate Like a Book* by Emily Dickinson on the power of the written word:

> *There is no Frigate like a Book*
> *To take us Lands away*
> *Nor any Coursers like a Page*
> *Of prancing Poetry –*
> *This Traverse may the poorest take*
> *Without oppress of Toll –*
> *How frugal is the Chariot*
> *That bears the Human Soul –*

Today I will remember that we are here to help each other and that I must be as ready to ask for help as to give it.

March 15th

On this day in 32 BC Julius Caesar, Roman general and politician, was assassinated. Famously told by soothsayers to 'Beware the Ides of March', Caesar nevertheless went to the Senate on that day where he was due to give a speech. He was met on the steps by the conspirators and stabbed, we are told, a total of 36 times.

The conspirators acted because they feared for the Roman Republic and democracy after Caesar had been proclaimed 'Dictator'. In fact their actions brought about the unforeseen result of ending the Republic, with the start of Imperial Rome.

Caesar had been highly popular with the Roman mob and in his will left lands and property to them. They were furious at his assassination and its perpetrators. Shakespeare recounted the events fairly correctly in his famous play.

Here is part of the speech by Marcus Antonius on Caesar's death:

> But yesterday the word of Caesar might
> Have stood against the world; now lies he there.
> And none so poor to do him reverence.
> O masters, if I were disposed to stir
> Your hearts and minds to mutiny and rage,
> I should do Brutus wrong, and Cassius wrong,
> Who, you all know, are honourable men:
> I will not do them wrong; I rather choose
> To wrong the dead, to wrong myself and you,
> Than I will wrong such honourable men.
> But here's a parchment with the seal of Caesar;
> I found it in his closet, 'tis his will:
> Let but the commons hear this testament –
> And they would go and kiss dead Caesar's wounds
> And dip their napkins in his sacred blood

Today I will try not to be a resentful person remembering past hurt; I will remind myself that by forgiving others, I am helping myself.

March 16th

On this day in 1951 American author Jack Kerouac was preparing to write his defining novel *On the Road*. The manuscript was to be typed on what he called 'the scroll' – a continuous, one hundred and twenty-foot scroll of tracing paper sheets that he carefully cut to size and taped together. His intention was that this roll would be fed continuously through his typewriter.

Thus Kerouac was planning the writing of a 'stream of consciousness' style of narrative, such as appears in James Joyce's *Ulysses*. Certainly he was a great admirer of Joyce; both *On the Road* and *Ulysses* are books about journeys, as indeed are so many great books.

Perhaps Kerouac knew this poem about riding down the road, Always Comes Evening, written by pulp fiction writer Robert E Howard who shot himself in 1936:

Riding down the road at evening with the stars or steed and shoon
I have heard an old man singing underneath a copper moon;
God, who gemmed with topaz twilights, opal portals of the day,
On our amaranthine mountains, why make human souls of clay?
For I rode the moon-mare's horses in the glory of my youth,
Wrestled with the hills at sunset – till I met brass-tinctured Truth.
Till I saw the temples topple, till I saw the idols reel,
Till my brain had turned to iron, and my heart had turned to steel.
Satan, Satan, brother Satan, fill my soul with frozen fire;
Feed with hearts of rose-white women ashes of my dead desire.
For my road runs out in thistles and my dreams have turned to dust.
And my pinions fade and falter to the raven wings of rust.
Riding down the road at evening when the wind was on the sea,
I have heard an old man singing, and he sang most drearily
Strange to hear, when dark lakes shimmer to the wailing of the loon,
Amethystine Homer singing under evening's copper moon.

Today I look for tolerance in others.

March 17th

On this day in AD 180 the Roman emperor and philosopher Marcus Aurelius died aged 58. He is chiefly remembered today for his philosophical writings as a follower of Stoicism.

His Meditations were initially addressed 'To Myself' and are a series of thoughts and observations for his own guidance and improvement, mainly on how to stay calm and focused in times of stress and turmoil.

Here is a poem on staying calm, *Hard Times*, by another deep thinker – Rabindranath Tagore:

Music is silenced, the dark descending slowly
Has stripped unending skies of all companions.
Weariness grips your limbs and within the locked horizons
Dumbly ring the bells of hugely gathering fears.
Still, O bird, O sightless bird,
Not yet, not yet the time to furl your wings.
It's not melodious woodlands but the leaps and falls
Of an ocean's drowsy booming,
Not a grove bedecked with flowers but a tumult flecked with foam.
Where is the shore that stored your buds and leaves?
Where the nest and the branch's hold?
But O my bird, O sightless bird,
Not yet, not yet the time to furl your wings.
All that is past: your fears and loves and hopes;
All that is lost: your words and lamentation;
No longer yours a home nor a bed composed of flowers.
For wings are all you have, and the sky's broadening courtyards,
And the dawn steeped in darkness, lacking all direction.
Dear bird, my sightless bird,
Not yet, not yet the time to furl your wings!

Today I will try to deal with all life's problems in a calm and sensible manner.

March 18th

On this day in 1314 the Grand Master of the Knights Templar, Jacques de Molay, was burnt to death at the stake, in Paris. The reason why this basically noble and gentle 72 year-old was so horribly put to death was that King Philip IV of France wanted to weaken the knights and take for himself the huge treasury that they possessed.

Since the fall of Acre in 1291 and the loss of the Holy Land, crusaders (which the Templars primarily were) had been out of fashion and countries like France saw such groups of armed warriors who had returned back in their territories as a threat. The Templars had been confident that the Pope would protect them from the trumped up charges of heresy put about by the King. No such thing happened.

Although some of the knights confessed to heresies under torture and were spared, de Molay and some others were sentenced to die. The old man met his death with dignity, though later it was said that at the end he had shouted out, summoning Philip IV and Pope Clement to meet him before God, where they would be judged for their crimes. Both men died within a year of de Molay – the old man's curse seemed to have worked. Here is Chaucer's description of a knight, from the *Canterbury Tales*:

> *A knight there was, and what a gentleman,*
> *Who, from the moment that he first began*
> *To ride about the world, loved chivalry,*
> *Truth, honour, freedom and all courtesy.*
> *Full worthy was he in his sovereign's war,*
> *And therein had he ridden, no man more,*
> *As well in Christendom as heathenesse,*
> *And honoured everywhere for worthiness.*
> *He was a truly perfect, noble knight.*

Today I will strive be strong enough to stand up for my beliefs, whatever the cost.

March 19th

On this day in 2008 British science fiction writer Sir Arthur C. Clarke died aged 90. A prolific writer, he is most famous for the screenplay of Stanley Kubrick's film: *2001 – A Space Odyssey*.

Clarke had an uncanny knack for predicting the future well in advance of events, thus he foresaw satellite communication and the universal use of computers for online banking and shopping, decades before they happened. Clarke was briefly married but openly gay and he spent the last 50 years of his life in Sri Lanka.

Here is a poem by James Weldon Johnson that reminds me of the film *2001 – A Space Odyssey*, despite being called *The Creation*:

> And God stepped out on space
> And he looked around and said,
> I'm lonely –
> I'll make me a world.
> And far as the eye of God could see
> Darkness covered everything,
> Blacker than a hundred midnights
> Down in a cypress swamp.
> Then God smiled,
> And the light broke
> And the darkness rolled up on one side
> And the light stood shining on the other,
> And God said "That's good!"
> Then God reached out and took the light in his hands,
> And God rolled the light around in his hands
> Until he made the sun

Today I am grateful for the wonder of the universe which is stranger than we may ever imagine; nevertheless we should not be afraid, because we are a part of it ourselves.

March 20th

On this day in 1828 Norwegian playwright Henrik Ibsen was born. Ibsen did not really achieve recognition until the play Peer Gynt appeared, by which time he was nearly 40. He produced a series of wonderful works including *The Wild Duck*, *A Doll's House* and *Hedda Gabler* which gained worldwide fame.

He is considered a modernist writer because of his realism and clear-eyed look at peoples' behaviours and their consequences. His topics, such as the ravages to a family caused by a father's venereal disease (Ghosts) were almost unbearable for Victorian audiences and caused considerable controversy. No wonder he is called the father of realism. He died at home, and his last words were 'on the contrary' – when he heard the nurse say he was feeling better. A realist to the last. This famous poem by Christina Rossetti is about saying goodbye:

> When I am dead, my dearest,
>   Sing no sad songs for me;
> Plant thou no roses at my head,
>   Nor shady cypress tree:
> Be the green grass above me
>   With showers and dewdrops wet;
> And if thou wilt, remember,
>   And if thou wilt, forget.
> I shall not see the shadows,
>   I shall not feel the rain;
> I shall not hear the nightingale
>   Sing on, as if in pain:
> And dreaming through the twilight
>   That doth not rise nor set,
> Haply I may remember,
>   And haply may forget.

Today I will stop making up plays and dramas for myself but I will concentrate on showing my real self and keeping it simple.

March 21st

On this day in 1685 the German composer Johann Sebastian Bach was born. One of music's all-time greats, Bach grew up in a musical household and struggled around the age of ten when his parents died.

Later, living with an elder brother, he was able to continue doing what he liked best – playing and composing music. During his life, Bach moved around the courts and cities of Northern Germany playing church organs and giving concerts. Some of his best known works are the Brandenburg concertos and his *Mass in B flat minor*. His influence on composers such as Mozart, Chopin, Schumann and Mendelssohn was enormous and Beethoven called him 'the original father of harmony'. Bach and Handel were born the same year, in the same part of Germany, but the two never met. Bach died aged 65.

Here is one of Shakespeare's lesser known sonnets, *VIII*, which rather nicely, suggests the pleasures of music:

> *Music to hear, why hear'st thou music sadly?*
> *Sweets with sweets war not, joy delights in joy.*
> *Why lov'st thou that which thou receiv'st not gladly,*
> *Or else receiv'st with pleasure thine annoy?*
> *If the true concord of well-tuned sounds,*
> *By unions married, do offend thine ear,*
> *They do but sweetly chide thee, who confounds*
> *In singleness the parts that thou shouldst bear.*
> *Mark how one string, sweet husband to another,*
> *Strikes each in each by mutual ordering,*
> *Resembling sire and child and happy mother*
> *Who all in one, one pleasing note do sing:*
> > *Whose speechless song, being many, seeming one,*
> > *Sings this to thee: "Thou single wilt prove none."*

Today I will remember the importance of keeping a balance and harmony in my life and I will work to make this happen.

March 22nd

On this day in 1941 American Poet Laureate Billy Collins was born. Called 'America's favourite poet' he has several best-selling volumes to his name. His poem *The Names* commemorates the victims of the 9/11 attacks.

His work is very contemporary and often presented as personal experience with considerable humour. For example: I Chop Some Parsley While Listening To Art Blakey's Version Of 'Three Blind Mice'. As an only child, he benefited greatly from the attention of his poetry loving mother who had the ability to remember and recite verses on almost any subject. Collins founded the Mid-Atlantic Review and teaches at several universities in the United States.

I think he would appreciate the immediacy of Katherine Mansfield's poems like this one, *Butterfly Laughter*:

> In the middle of our porridge plates
> There was a blue butterfly painted
> And each morning we tried who should reach the
>   butterfly first.
> Then the Grandmother said: "Do not eat the poor
>   butterfly."
> That made us laugh.
> Always she said it and always it started us laughing.
> It seemed such a sweet little joke.
> I was certain that one fine morning
> The butterfly would fly out of our plates,
> Laughing the teeniest laugh in the world,
> And perch on the Grandmother's lap.

Today I ask no more than to be able to savour life's delicious moments with gratitude.

March 23rd

On this day in 1901 Dame Nellie Melba revealed the secret of her famous toast. The toast had been invented along with the dessert Peach Melba in her honour by the famous French chef, Escoffier.

Melba was an Australian whose voice was universally acclaimed as one of the most beautiful there has ever been. She acquired a huge following, especially at Covent Garden. She adopted the name Melba (a shortened version of Melbourne, her home town). Some critics felt that her repertoire was too small and limited and criticised her willingness to sing secondary roles and mere folk songs at times. On the other hand, she called their attitude 'artistic snobbery'.

Here is the lovely folk song *Comin though the Rye* by Robert Burns, that she recorded so beautifully:

Gin a body meet a body
Comin through the rye
Gin a body kiss a body
Need a body cry?
Chorus:
Ilka lassie has her laddie
Nane, they say, hae I
Yet aa the lads they smile at me
When comin through the rye.
Gin a body meet a body
Comin through the toon,
Gin a body greet a body
Need a body froon?
Amang the train there is a
swain

I dearly loe masel
But what's his name an where's
   his hame
I dinna care to tell
Gin a body meet a body
Comin frae the well
Gin a body kiss a body
Need a body tell?
Ilka lassie has her laddie
Nane, they say, hae I
Yet aa the lads they smile at me
When comin through the rye.

Today I ask for the courage to address and to change where necessary, the things that I need to address today.

March 24th

On this day in 1909 Irish playwright and poet John Millington Synge died. Many of his best known plays are about Irish Catholic peasants in the west of Ireland. Performances of *The Playboy of the Western World* were interrupted by disturbances at the Abbey theatre in Dublin, with people objecting to a perceived slight on the noble peasantry.

Synge lived in Paris and London at times and was a big influence on later Irish writers such as Beckett and O'Casey; it is said that the tramps and vagabonds that feature in many of Beckett's plays were copied from his work. Synge died at the untimely age of 38.

This poem, *The Curse*, was written about the sister of an author's enemy who disapproved of *The Playboy of the Western World*:

> *Lord, confound this surly sister,*
> *Blight her brow with blotch and blister,*
> *Cramp her larynx, lung, and liver,*
> *In her guts a galling give her.*
> *Let her live to earn her dinners*
> *In Mountjoy with seedy sinners:*
> *Lord, this judgment quickly bring,*
> *And I'm your servant, J. M. Synge.*

Today I will try to grow spiritually by replacing fear and hatred with faith.

March 25th

On this day in 1881 the novelist Mary Webb was born. Brought up in Shropshire, her stories are reminiscent in plot and style of her better known counterpart, Thomas Hardy. Her rustic heroes and heroines speaking mostly in local dialect, bringing a realism to the books that was not always matched by the sentimental and sometimes fanciful story lines.

In spite of the misery and poverty and despair that they often contained, her books acquired a large following in the 1930s – especially after the British Prime Minister Stanley Baldwin referred to her in a speech as a 'neglected genius'.

Not everyone was a fan, however, and her work inspired Stella Gibbons to write the much loved parody *Cold Comfort Farm*, based on Webb's *Precious Bane*. Gibbons later said: "The large agonised faces in Mary Webb's book annoyed me ... I did not believe people were any more despairing in Herefordshire than in Camden Town". Here is a poem by Mary Webb, *Treasures*:

Into the scented woods we'll go
And see the blackthorn swim in snow.
High above, in the budding leaves,
A brooding dove awakes and grieves;
The glades with mingled music stir,
And wildly laughs the woodpecker.
When blackthorn petals pearl the breeze,
There are the twisted hawthorn trees
Thick-set with buds, as clear and pale
As golden water or green hail –
As if a storm of rain had stood
Enchanted in the thorny wood,
And, hearing fairy voices call,
Hung poised, forgetting how to fall.

Today I will be mindful of the beauty in nature and all things around me.

March 26th

On this day in 1930 American poet Gregory Corso was born. He was a member of the Beat Generation and a particular friend of Allen Ginsberg. Despite a spell in prison and a poor education, he was able to charm his way into Harvard. Corso saw poetry as coming from the heart, through inspiration, and along the way was prepared to disdain and disrespect everything except the poetry itself.

His ashes, at his request, are buried in Rome at the foot of Percy Shelley's grave in a touching tribute to the man he admired as a 'revolutionary of spirit'. Here is a poem by Canadian Bliss Carman whose work is not as well-known as Corso's but has a similar introspective feel, *A Fireside Vision*:

> *Once I walked the world enchanted*
> *Through the scented woods of spring,*
> *Hand in hand with Love, in rapture*
> *Just to hear a bluebird sing.*
> *Now the lonely winds of autumn*
> *Moan about my gusty eaves,*
> *As I sit beside the fire*
> *Listening to the flying leaves.*
> *As the dying embers settle*
> *And the twilight falls apace,*
> *Through the gloom I see a vision*
> *Full of ardour, full of grace.*
> *Eyes more wonderful than evening.*
> *With the new moon on the hill,*
> *Mouth with traces of God's humour*
> *In its corners lurking still.*
> *Ah, she smiles, in recollection;*
> *Lays a hand upon my brow;*
> *Rests this head upon Love's bosom!*
> *Surely it is April now*

Today I give thanks for the poetic revolutionaries of spirit.

March 27th

On this day in 1886 the German-American architect Mies van der Rohe was born. One of the founders of modernistic architecture, together with Le Corbusier and Lloyd Wright, he became the last director of the Bauhaus School before it was forced to close by the Nazis.

Mies devised architecture that was based on framework and open spaces, and originated phrases such as 'less is good' and 'God is in the details'.

Today's poem by Will Allen Dromgoole is of building, *The Bridge Builder*:

An old man going a lone highway,
Came, at the evening cold and gray,
To a chasm vast and deep and wide.
Through which was flowing a sullen tide
The old man crossed in the twilight dim,
The sullen stream had no fear for him;
But he turned when safe on the other side
And built a bridge to span the tide.
"Old man," said a fellow pilgrim near,
"You are wasting your strength with building here;
Your journey will end with the ending day,
You never again will pass this way;
You've crossed the chasm, deep and wide,
Why build this bridge at evening tide?"
The builder lifted his old gray head;
"Good friend, in the path I have come," he said,
"There followed after me to-day
A youth whose feet must pass this way.
This chasm that has been as naught to me
To that fair-haired youth may a pitfall be;
He, too, must cross in the twilight dim;
Good friend, I am building this bridge for him!

Today I will work at building my life carefully and cleanly.

March 28th

On this day in 1757 the unsuccessful regicide Robert-François Damiens was executed. Damiens was a simple man from Arras who attacked the French King Louis XV, inflicting a superficial wound. For this perceived heinous crime, he was sentenced to be drawn and quartered in the Place de Grève, Paris. On the morning of his execution he said 'la journée sera rude' (today will be tough) and he was right. After first being tortured with red hot pincers he was then pulled apart by four horses attached to his arms and legs; his truncated body was finally burnt at the stake. This appalling event, viewed by thousands, may have led to some of the dreadful cruelties that occurred later during the Revolution. Maximilien Robespierre, infamous for the 1793 'Reign of Terror', also came from Arras. The horror of Damiens' death is reminiscent of the grimness found sometimes in a Greek tragedy. Here is an excerpt from Aeschylus' *Oresteia*, where Electra is speaking about the murder of her father, Agamemnon and revenge:

> *What they did to his body*
> *They did to my spirit and heart.*
> *They flung him out like a dead dog*
> *To rot in the sun.*
> *If Agamemnon's severed head could have sobbed,*
> *That was how I laughed.*
> *Insane with grief.*
> *If you want to know what grief means*
> *Remember me.*
> *Chorus: Now let your will, like your grief,*
> *Be stronger than life.*
> *The past is stronger than life –*
> *Nothing can alter it.*

Today I will try to face each day with courage. Some days will be tough, but not as tough as this day was for Robert-François Damiens.

March 29th

On this day in 1957 the Anglo Irish writer Joyce Cary died. Cary originally wanted to be a painter but realised that he would never be top rank and decided to write instead. Some of his books are about life in an Ireland that was left behind when his family moved to London when he was young.

He spent time abroad, especially in Africa, which featured in several of his books. His most famous novel is *The Horse's Mouth*, a story of a fictional artist's life that was made into a film. He died aged 68 after a long struggle with motor neurone disease.

Cary contracted motor neurone disease and must have longed for the peaceful living depicted in this poem, *The Lake Isle of Innisfree*, by William Butler Yeats, another Irishman:

> *I will arise and go now, and go to Innisfree,*
> *And a small cabin build there, of clay and wattles made:*
> *Nine bean-rows will I have there, a hive for the honey-bee;*
> *And live alone in the bee-loud glade.*
> *And I shall have some peace there,*
> *for peace comes dropping slow,*
> *Dropping from the veils of the morning*
> *to where the cricket sings;*
> *There midnight's all a glimmer, and noon a purple glow,*
> *And evening full of the linnet's wings.*
> *I will arise and go now, for always night and day*
> *I hear lake water lapping with low sounds by the shore;*
> *While I stand on the roadway, or on the pavements grey,*
> *I hear it in the deep heart's core.*

Today I will try to respect all people and remember that anger and resentment can only harm me.

March 30th

On this day in 1853 the Dutch painter Vincent Van Gogh was born. A recent biography suggested that his death at the age of 37 was not suicide but an accident caused by two local boys playing cowboys with a faulty gun. The painter had been in mental torment with large mood swings for a long time. Great paintings do not have to come from great emotional upheaval but, in the case of Van Gogh, the two are hard to separate because his feelings were so involved in the painting process. Whereas other artists such as Monet, for example, painted what they saw, Van Gogh painted what he felt about what he saw.

There is something infinitely moving about the thought of this lonely and unstable genius channelling his emotional ups and downs onto beautiful canvasses which few people appreciated until after he died. It is what makes him so special. Here is Baudelaire's famous poem on loneliness – he knew about it too:

> *What will you say tonight, poor lonely soul,*
> *What will you say old withered heart of mine,*
> *To the most beautiful, the best, most dear,*
> *Whose heavenly regard brings back your bloom?*
> *We will assign our pride to sing her praise:*
> *Nothing excels the sweetness of her will;*
> *Her holy body has an angel's scent,*
> *Her eye invests us with a cloak of light.*
> *Whether it be in night and solitude,*
> *Or in the streets among the multitude,*
> *Her ghost before us dances like a torch.*
> *It speaks out: 'I am lovely and command*
> *That you will love only the Beautiful;*
> *I am your Guardian, Madonna, Muse!*

Today I ask that I will never be so lonely that I find it unbearable; I will not be too proud to ask for help.

March 31st

O n this day in 1621 the English poet Andrew Marvell was born. He was a clever and educated man who managed successfully to steer his way through the difficult times of the Civil War, Cromwell and the restoration of King Charles II.

As a close friend of Milton he was also able to protect the blind poet from any retribution by the restored King – Milton had shown himself as anti-monarchy during the Commonwealth.

Here is one of his poems that shows his awareness of the dangerous times that he lived in, *A Garden, Written After The Civil Wars*:

> See how the flowers, as at parade,
> Under their colours stand display'd:
> Each regiment in order grows,
> That of the tulip, pink, and rose.
> But when the vigilant patrol
> Of stars walks round about the pole,
> Their leaves that to the stalks are curl'd,
> Seem to their staves the ensigns furl'd.
> Then in some flower's beloved hut
> Each bee, as sentinel, is shut,
> And sleeps so too; but if once stirr'd,
> She runs you through, nor asks the word.
> What luckless apple did we taste
> To make us mortal and thee waste!
> Unhappy! Shall we never more
> That sweet militia restore,
> When gardens only had their towers,
> And all the garrisons were flowers;
> When roses only arms might bear,
> And men did rosy garlands wear.

Today I will work towards the goal of a world free from fear.

April 1st

On this day people like to play tricks on each other. Nobody knows why – perhaps that's what the attraction is. It seems to have started in the 19th century.

In France they call it 'Poisson d'Avril' (April Fish); again nobody knows why, or cares too much. So we go on, year after year. It may not be especially fun, but it's better than April 5th (start of the tax year in the UK). Here is part of a jolly poem, *April Fool's Day*, that was sent to a newspaper in 1900 by a WE Cowles, about whom nothing is known:

> *Talk about yer Chris'masses*
> *Fourth o' Julys and cirkusses –*
> *They ain't in it for the real fun*
> *That's to be had on April one;*
> *Even Hallowe'en is very tame*
> *To April first – that is 'f yer game.*
> *I think that April first must be*
> *Ind'pendence Day fer kids like me,*
> *When we kin play all sorts of jokes*
> *And not be punished by our folks –*
> *Though pa, he says, in a threat'nin' way:*
> *"Bill, no nonsense from you today!"*
> *The teacher has her troubles too*
> *(You know what mischeevous boys can do).*
> *But when I hollered "April Fool!"*
> *She kept me in long after school.*
> *Say, you look as though you might*
> *Know how a boy'd feel at night,*
> *As though a big day's work was done,*
> *And how h'd fooled 'em all –'cept one –*
> *For pa, he'd said to me, one side,*
> *"Don't ye fool Me, 'r I'll tan yer hide!"*

Today I will remember: fun is fun, reality is reality.

April 2nd

On this day in 1840 the French author Émile Zola was born. He was a prolific writer of novels, the best known being *Thérèse Raquin* and *Germinal*. Brought up in Provence and a friend of Cézanne, he travelled to Paris with the painter and soon achieved success.

His moment of true glory came during the notorious Dreyfus affair when he wrote an open letter, published in *L'Aurore*, with the famous headline 'J'Accuse', an indictment of the French government's anti-Semitic attitude. After this he was prosecuted and fled briefly to England before returning to a pardon. Zola and his wife Alexandrine died of carbon monoxide poisoning, perhaps caused by a faulty chimney. He was 62. Years later, a chimney sweep is said to have confessed to blocking the chimney for political reasons, but nothing was proved. This poem, *My Books* is by Stéphane Mallarmé, a contemporary of Zola's:

> *My books closed again on Paphos' name,*
> *It delights me to choose with solitary genius*
> *A ruin, by foam-flecks in thousands blessed*
> *Beneath hyacinth, far off, in days of fame.*
> *Let the cold flow with its silence of scythes,*
> *I'll not ululate here in a 'no' that's empty*
> *If this frolic so white near the ground denies*
> *To each site the honour of false scenery.*
> *My hunger regaled by no fruits here I see*
> *Finds equal taste in their learned deficiency:*
> *Let one burst with human fragrance and flesh!*
> *While my love pokes the fire, foot on cold iron*
> *I brood for a long time perhaps with distress*
> *On the other's seared breast of an ancient Amazon.*

Today I will remember that actions have consequences but that inaction also has consequences. I ask for the wisdom to make the right choices.

April 3rd

On this day in 1783, the year when America's War of Independence ended, the writer Washington Irving was born. He was named after America's greatest statesman. Irving grew up in Manhattan and is best known for his stories of American folklore such as *Rip van Winkle* and T*he Legend of Sleepy Hollow.*

Irving is held to be the first American man of letters, meaning the first to earn a living through his own writing. He also performed diplomatic roles while in Europe, some of which gave him material for his stories. He never married but was generally recognised as a charming and witty guest, popular with the ladies.

Here is a typical poem of his, *A Certain Young Lady*:

> There's a certain young lady,
> Who's just in her heyday,
>   And full of all mischief, I ween;
> So teasing! So pleasing!
> Capricious! Delicious!
>   And you know very well whom I mean.
> With a stately step – such as
> You'd expect in a duchess –
>   And a brow might distinguish a queen,
> With a mighty proud air,
> That says "touch me who dare,"
>   And you know very well whom I mean.
> Heaven help the adorer
> Who happens to bore her,
>   The lover who wakens her spleen;
> But too blest for a sinner
> Is he who shall win her,
>   And you know very well whom I mean.

Today I will try to learn from the example of others and recognise how they achieve serenity.

April 4th

On this day in 1774 the poet, novelist and playwright Oliver Goldsmith died aged 43. Born in Ireland, he went to Trinity College, Dublin and later studied medicine, unsuccessfully, in Edinburgh. He moved to London and began writing, his most famous works being the play *She Stoops to Conquer* and the novel *The Vicar of Wakefield*.

Goldsmith was always short of money because he was a compulsive gambler. A founder member of 'The Club', a literary group that included Dr Samuel Johnson and Horace Walpole, he was known as the 'inspired idiot' because of his dissolute lifestyle.

Johnson wrote this epitaph: "Oliver Goldsmith: A Poet, Naturalist, and Historian, who left scarcely any style of writing untouched, and touched nothing that he did not adorn. Of all the passions, whether smiles were to move or tears, a powerful yet gentle master. In genius, vivid, versatile, sublime. In style, clear, elevated, elegant."

Here is one of Oliver Goldsmith's poems, *The Gift (To Iris)*:

Say, cruel Iris, pretty rake,
Dear mercenary beauty,
What annual offering shall I make,
Expressive of my duty?
My heart, a victim to thine eyes,
Should I at once deliver,
Say, would the angry fair one prize
The gift, who slights the giver?
A bill, a jewel, watch, or toy,
My rivals give – and let 'em;
If gems, or gold, impart a joy,
I'll give them-when I get 'em.

I'll give-but not the full-blown rose,
Or rose-bud more in fashion;
Such short-liv'd offerings but disclose
A transitory passion.
I'll give thee something yet unpaid,
Not less sincere, than civil:
I'll give thee-ah! Too charming maid,
I'll give thee-to the devil

Today I reflect that there is a time to be foolish and a time to be serious.

April 5th

On this day in 1837 the poet Algernon Charles Swinburne was born. Swinburne was a well-born and clever young man who did well at Oxford and was able to live a fairly leisured life. He spent much of his childhood, when not at school, in Northumbria which he regarded as his spiritual home. Poems such as *Grace Darling* are about this area of the country.

He was a well-liked member of the Pre-Raphaelite circle and his poetry was considered daring at the time, especially his homage to lesbianism and homosexuality. A rebellious and excitable figure, his alcoholism eventually got the better of him and he spent the last 30 years of his life living quietly and writing little, in the care of Theodore Watts – a close friend and doctor in Putney.

It was said of Watts that he saved the man but killed the poet. Swinburne was also an algolagniac (one who derives sexual pleasure and arousal from physical pain) and this shows in some of his poetry:

> There was a graven image of Desire
> Painted with red blood on a ground of gold
> Passing between the young men and the old,
> And by him Pain, whose body shone like fire,
> And Pleasure with gaunt hands that grasped their hire.
> Of his left wrist, with fingers clenched and cold,
> The insatiable Satiety kept hold,
> Walking with feet unshod that pashed the mire.
> The senses and the sorrows and the sins,
> And the strange loves that suck the breasts of Hate
> Till lips and teeth bite in their sharp indenture,
> Followed like beasts with flap of wings and fins.
> Death stood aloof behind a gaping grate,
> Upon whose lock was written Peradventure.

Today I remember that I seek spiritual progress not spiritual perfection.

April 6th

On this day in 1947 American playwright and Pulitzer Prize winner Arthur Miller won a Tony award for his play *All My Sons*. Miller was married four times including to the film idol Marilyn Monroe. His life was also defined by his battle with Congress's Communist-hunting Un-American Activities Committee. He steadfastly refused to give any names of people suspected of Communist sympathies. He afterwards wrote *The Crucible* about the Salem witch hunts, as a parody of the persecution that he had undergone.

Here are some lines from *Antigone*, Sophocles' great play about Antigone, daughter of Oedipus, who bravely died for her principles:

> King Creon: Didst thou, then, dare to disobey these laws
> Antigone: Yes, for it was not Zeus who gave them forth,
> Nor Justice, dwelling with the Gods below,
> Who traced these laws for all the sons of men;
> Nor did I deem thy edicts strong enough,
> Coming from mortal man, to set at naught
> The unwritten laws of God that know not change.
> They are not of to-day nor yesterday,
> But live for ever, nor can man assign
> When first they sprang to being. Not through fear
> Of any man's resolve was I prepared
> Before the Gods to bear the penalty
> Of sinning against these. That I should die
> I knew (how should I not?), though thy decree
> Had never spoken. And, before my time
> If I should die, I reckon this a gain;
> For whoso lives, as I, in many woes,
> How can it be but death shall bring him gain?
> And so for me to bear this doom of thine has nothing painful.

Today I reflect on the strength of those who stand up for their beliefs.

April 7th

On this day in 1770 the English poet William Wordsworth was born. A career poet who became Poet Laureate in his later years, Wordsworth is always linked to the Lake District. His famous definition of poetry is still often quoted: "the spontaneous overflow of powerful feelings: it takes its origin from emotion recollected in tranquillity."

He travelled extensively throughout Germany and visited revolutionary France in 1791 which impressed him greatly. He fell in love with a French girl and fathered a daughter, both of whom he supported as best he could for the rest of his life. It was his friendship with the poet Samuel Taylor Coleridge that was to further his career, with the publication of Lyrical Ballads to which they both contributed.

This established them as leaders of the 'Romantic Movement'. Wordsworth married Mary Hutchinson, his childhood sweetheart, in 1802 though his sister Dorothy continued to live with them.

Here is a Wordsworth poem, *Lucy*, that fits his definition of poetry:

> She dwelt among th' untrodden ways
> Beside the springs of Dove,
> A Maid whom there were none to praise
> And very few to love.
> A Violet by a mossy stone
> Half-hidden from the Eye!
> – Fair, as a star when only one
> Is shining in the sky!
> She liv'd unknown, and few could know
> When Lucy ceas'd to be;
> But she is in her Grave, and Oh!
> The difference to me.

Today I will remember that this day is all I have – yesterday is gone and tomorrow may never happen.

April 8th

On this day in AD 750 the Chinese poet Du Fu was writing verse. Possibly China's greatest poet, he was born during the Tang Dynasty and lived simply but much of his writing still resonates today. Here is part of his poem about the preparations for war, *The Song of the Wagons*:

The wagons rumble and roll, the horses whinny and neigh,
The conscripts each have bows and arrows at their waists.
Their parents, wives and children run to see them off,
So much dust's stirred up, it hides the Xianyang Bridge.
They pull clothes, stamp their feet and, weeping, bar the way,
The weeping voices rise straight up and strike the clouds.
A passer-by at the roadside asks a conscript why,
The conscript answers only that drafting happens often.
At fifteen, many were sent north to guard the river,
Even at forty, they had to till fields in the west.
When we went away, the elders bound our heads,
Returning with heads white, we're sent back off to the frontier.
At the border posts, shed blood becomes a sea,
The martial emperor's dream of expansion has no end.
Have you not seen the two hundred districts east of the mountains,
Where thorns and brambles grow in countless hamlets?
Although an elder can ask me this, how can a soldier dare to
    complain, even in this winter time?
Soldiers from west of the pass keep moving.
The magistrate is eager for taxes, but how can we afford to pay?

Today I will remember that I cannot live alone; I cannot do it all myself; I must recognise the need for help and not be too proud to ask for it.

April 9th

On this day in 1806 the engineer and designer Isambard Kingdom Brunel was born. His works, such as the *Great Western Railway*, and his numerous bridges and tunnels are still in use today. He also designed iron propeller-driven steamships that made safe transatlantic crossings possible.

It was Brunel's dream to extend travel on the Great Western Railway as far as America. By this he meant that travellers could purchase a ticket in London, travel by rail to Wales and there embark on a steamship and continue to New York. In 1836 this became a reality. He married and had children but died of a stroke at the relatively young age of 53; he had always been a heavy smoker and was often photographed with a cigar. Here is a poem by William Blake, a bit of a Luddite, who died when Brunel was 21, *I see the Four-fold Man*:

> I see the Four-fold Man, The Humanity in deadly sleep
> And it's fallen Emanation, the Spectre and its cruel Shadow.
> I see the Past, Present and Future existing all at once
> Before me. O Divine Spirit, sustain me on thy wings,
> That I may awake Albion from his long and cold repose;
> For Bacon and Newton, sheath'd in dismal steel, their terrors hang
> Like iron scourges over Albion: reasonings like vast serpents
> Infold around my limbs, bruising my minute articulations.
> I turn my eyes to the schools and universities of Europe
> And there behold the Loom of Locke, whose Woof rages dire,
> Wash'd by the Water-wheels of Newton: black the cloth
> In heavy wreaths folds over every nation: cruel works
> Of many Wheels I view, wheel without wheel, with cogs tyrannic
> Moving by compulsion each other, not as those in Eden, which,
> Wheel within wheel, in freedom revolve in harmony and peace.

Today I ask that I will recognise the inevitability of change while respecting the legacy of the past.

April 10th

On this day in 1829 William Booth, founder of the Salvation Army, was born. After years of work as a travelling Methodist preacher who was trying to help the poor, Booth one day realised that he and his helpers were a kind of army. He began to organise them on military lines, naming himself as General and giving others appropriate ranks and uniforms. He adapted popular songs into strident marching songs, giving them Christian themes so 'the devil should not have all the best tunes'. Within a few years the Salvation Army was a worldwide 'brand' and it thrives today, doing an enormous amount of good work. When Booth died in 1912, aged 83, forty Salvation Army bands and ten thousand Christian soldiers marched behind his coffin.

This poem was written by Vachel Lindsay on the occasion, *Above the Battle's Front*:

> St. Francis, Buddha, Tolstoi, and St. John –
> Friends, if you four, as pilgrims, hand in hand,
> Returned, the hate of earth once more to dare,
> And walked upon the water and the land,
> If you, with words celestial, stopped these kings
> For sober conclave, ere their battle great,
> Would they for one deep instant then discern
> Their crime, their heart-rot, and their fiend's estate?
> If you should float above the battle's front,
> Pillars of cloud, of fire that does not slay,
> Bearing a fifth within your regal train,
> The Son of David in his strange array –
> If, in his majesty, he towered toward Heaven,
> Would they have hearts to see or understand?

Today I remember with gratitude the work of William Booth and his army; I will do my best to help those less fortunate than myself.

April 11th

On this day in 2007 American author and artist Kurt Vonnegut Junior died, aged 84. Vonnegut smoked untipped cigarettes most of his adult life, sardonically calling the habit 'a classy way to commit suicide'. In fact he died after falling down the stairs at home.

Captured by the Germans during World War II, he witnessed the bombing of Dresden while imprisoned there in a slaughterhouse. It turned him into a lifelong pacifist and humanist. Vonnegut's writing is a mixture of autobiography, humour, satire and science fiction. *The New York Times* called him "the counterculture's novelist."

His novels *Cat's Cradle* and *Slaughterhouse Five* are regarded as some of the best works by an American writer in the 20th century. He was a great admirer of Mark Twain whose ironic poems he must have enjoyed.

Here is part of one:

> *O Lord, our father,*
> *Our young patriots, idols of our hearts,*
> *Go forth to battle – be Thou near them!*
> *With them, in spirit, we also go forth*
> *From the sweet peace of our beloved firesides to smite the*
> *foe.*
> *O Lord, our God,*
> *Help us to tear their soldiers*
> *To bloody shreds with our shells;*
> *Help us to lay waste their humble homes*
> *With a hurricane of fire;*
> *We ask it in the spirit of love –*
> *Of Him who is the source of love,*
> *And who is the ever-faithful*
> *Refuge and Friend of all that are sore beset and seek His*
> *aid with humble and contrite hearts. Amen*

Today I will work towards the goal of peace in the world.

April 12th

On this day in 1961 the Russian cosmonaut Yuri Gagarin became the first man in space when he orbited the earth. Gagarin's small size of 5ft 2in meant that he could fit in the tiny Vostok space capsule but he must have had other qualities, as all but three of his fellow cosmonauts voted for him to be 'the one'. He seems to have been a genuinely nice and humble man.

After his great feat, he travelled to many countries and liked to meet ordinary people. Tragically, he died aged 34 in an aircraft accident that seems to have happened through botched flight control information; the Soviets didn't always get things right.

Here is a poem by Wordsworth about the stars that Gagarin saw:

> It is no Spirit who from heaven hath flown,
> And is descending on his embassy;
> Nor Traveller gone from earth the heavens to espy!
> 'Tis Hesperus – there he stands with glittering crown,
> First admonition that the sun is down!
> O most ambitious Star! An inquest wrought
> Within me when I recognised thy light;
> A moment I was startled at the sight:
> And, while I gazed, there came to me a thought
> That I might step beyond my natural race
> As thou seem'st now to do; might one day trace
> Some ground not mine; and, strong her strength above,
> My Soul, an Apparition in the place,
> Tread there with steps that no one shall reprove!

Today I will remember the words of Oscar Wilde: 'we are all in the gutter but some of us are looking at the stars'.

April 13th

On this day in 1906 the poet and playwright Samuel Beckett was born. Beckett was a surprisingly good cricketer who earned himself an entry in Wisden, the cricket lovers' bible – the only Nobel laureate to do so. In his forties he realised that he must concentrate on minimalism. His most famous play *Waiting for Godot*, which appeared in 1953, certainly followed this idea. The critic Vivian Mercier wrote that he "has achieved a theoretical impossibility – a play in which nothing happens, that yet keeps audiences glued to their seats." Beckett was very well educated and was influenced by Greek tragedy (where much happens); it was the simple structure that he liked. From this taste, in Sophocles' *Oedipus Rex*, did waiting for Creon inspire *Waiting for Godot*?

Oedipus:

My poor children! I know you well and I know your pain.
I know very well that you are all gripped by despair.
Yet no one is in greater pain than I am because your pain affects
*   only you, each one of you, alone, whereas I ache for the whole*
*   city and for all of you. So have no fear, I'm not asleep. I am wide*
*   awake to your misfortune. My soul cries for us all.*
I have lost many tears and have travelled many paths of thought
*   to find a way out of this until, finally, I have decided to put into*
*   action the only possible solution that came to my mind:*
I have sent Creon, my wife's brother, Menoikeos' son, to Apollo's
*   oracle to ask what we should do to save our city; to find out what*
*   deed or what word should we do or say to save our country.*
In fact, Creon should have returned by now and I'm beginning to
*   worry. Let him come and tell us what needs to be done.*
Then I would indeed be a terrible man if I did not do all that the god
*   asks! (They all look into the distance and see Creon*
approaching.)

Today I will remember the benefits of minimalism although I will be careful not to miss the important things in life.

April 14th

On this day in 1939 the classic American novel *The Grapes of Wrath* by John Steinbeck was published. The brutal realism of the Joad family's epic journey from the Depression-hit Oklahoma dust bowl to California and the troubles that they endure, make this a hard but unforgettable story.

It is Steinbeck's J'Accuse and his masterpiece which he promoted saying: "I want to put a tag of shame on the greedy bastards who are responsible for this (the Great Depression)". *The Grapes of Wrath* is regularly listed among the 100 greatest novels in the English language.

Steinbeck won the Nobel Prize for Literature and died in 1968, aged 66. Apparently he never doubted that he would be a great writer.

Here is a poem about poverty – *Holy Thursday* by William Blake:

> Is this a holy thing to see,
> In a rich and fruitful land,
> Babes reduced to misery,
> Fed with cold and usurous hand?
> Is that trembling cry a song?
> Can it be a song of joy?
> And so many children poor?
> It is a land of poverty!
> And their sun does never shine.
> And their fields are bleak & bare.
> And their ways are fill'd with thorns.
> It is eternal winter there.
> For where-e'er the sun does shine,
> And where-e'er the rain does fall:
> Babe can never hunger there,
> Nor poverty the mind appall.

Today I will remember that it is better to give than to receive.

April 15th

On this day in 1912 the transatlantic steamship Titanic sank after hitting an iceberg One of the greatest peacetime maritime disasters, around 1500 people perished. The losses were made worse by the inadequate number of lifeboats, with provision for only 1178 people of the 2224 on board.

Another factor was the near freezing water. Nearby ships might have been able to help more but seemed curiously unmoved by the distress rockets that they saw. Perhaps nobody could believe that such a great vessel could really be in difficulty.

Only the Carpathia, a fellow White Star liner, gave wholehearted assistance and took on board over seven hundred survivors. The wreck of the Titanic was discovered in 1985 lying at about 12,000ft on the ocean floor. Many objects have been salvaged over the years and put on display, but the wreckage is too fragile to be raised and continues to deteriorate.

Here is a poem about the sinking, by Thomas Hardy:

In a solitude of the sea
Deep from human vanity,
And the Pride of Life that planned her, stilly couches she.
Steel chambers, late the pyres
Of her salamandrine fires,
Cold currents thrid, and turn to rhythmic tidal lyres.
Over the mirrors meant
To glass the opulent
The sea-worm crawls – grotesque, slimed, dumb, indifferent.
Jewels in joy designed
To ravish the sensuous mind
Lie lightless, all their sparkles bleared and black and blind

Today I ask that I will be able to handle whatever problems happen today, large or small.

April 16th

On this day in 1787 the first play by an American writer was performed at the John Street Theatre in New York City. Entitled *The Contrast*, by Royall Tyler, it was a comedy that satirised Americans who followed British fashions (the War of Independence was a recent memory).

The play can thus be seen as the start of the great theatrical tradition and industry, now known as Broadway. In 2014 over 13 million people paid 1.3 billion dollars to watch Broadway shows. The influence of American drama and musicals continues to be immense. It seems that we have had a constant taste for live drama since the time of Sophocles and Euripides in ancient Greece over two thousand years ago. Long may it last.

Here is a fragment of a Sophocles play from the fifth century BC, about the effect that love has upon us – it is just as relevant today:

When ice appears out of doors
And boys seize it while it is solid,
At first they experience new pleasures.
But in the end their pride
Will not allow them to let it go,
But their discovery is not good for them
If it stays in their hands.
In exactly the same way desire
Drives lovers to act and not to act

Today I reflect on the power that the immediacy of live drama has to teach us truths about ourselves.

April 17th

On this day in 1397 Geoffrey Chaucer recounted the *Canterbury Tales* at the court of King Richard II of England. The *Canterbury Tales* put him at the forefront of writers in mediaeval England.

The collection of tales from members of the little pilgrim band riding slowly from London to Canterbury is unforgettable. He also held several official posts and may have made enemies; there are even theories that he was murdered as a result. Chaucer is the first author to be buried in Poet's Corner at Westminster Abbey.

Here is one of his poems, *Merciless Beauty (Merciles Beaute)*:

> *Your eyes two whole slay me suddenly;*
> *I may the beauty of them not sustain*
> *So wounds it, throughout my heart keen.*
> *Unless your word will heal, all hastily,*
> *My heart's wound while it is yet green,*
>   *Your eyes two whole slay me suddenly;*
>   *I may the beauty of them not sustain.*
> *By my truth, I tell you faithfully*
> *That you are of my life and death the queen,*
> *For at my death the truth shall be seen:*
>   *Your eyes two whole slay me suddenly;*
>   *I may the beauty of them not sustain,*
>   *So wounds it throughout my heart keen.*
> *So has your beauty from your heart chased*
> *Pity, that it avails not to complain,*
> *For Pride holds your mercy by a chain.*
> *Though guiltless, my death you have purchased.*
> *I tell you truly, needing not to feign,*
>   *So has your beauty from your heart chased*
>   *Pity, that it avails not to complain*

Today I will remember that we cannot receive unless we give.

April 18th

On this day in 1955 the Swiss physicist Albert Einstein died of an aneurism, aged 76. He could have had surgery but refused, saying: "I want to go when I want. It is tasteless to prolong life artificially. I have done my share, it is time to go. I will do it elegantly."

His Theory of Relativity is considered one of the biggest advances ever made in science but he remained a humble person. Some of his sayings are difficult to understand. What did he really mean by saying: 'God does not play dice with the world'?

This part of a poem by Shelley has a rather simpler view of the heavens, *Ode to Heaven*:

> *Palace-roof of cloudless nights?*
> *Paradise of golden lights!*
> *Deep, immeasurable, vast,*
> *Which art now, and which wert then!*
> *Of the Present and the Past,*
> *Of the eternal Where and When,*
> *Presence-chamber, temple, home,*
> *Ever-canopying dome,*
> *Of acts and ages yet to come!*
> *Glorious shapes have life in thee,*
> *Earth, and all earth's company;*
> *Living globes which ever throng*
> *Thy deep chasms and wildernesses;*
> *And green worlds that glide along;*
> *And swift stars with flashing tresses;*
> *And icy moons most cold and bright,*
> *And mighty suns beyond the night,*
> *Atoms of intensest light.*

Today I recognise that spirituality is the 'something different' that has been missing for many of us.

April 19th

On this day in 1989 a pro-democracy student rally began in Tiananmen Square, Beijing. Popular support for the rally grew rapidly and there were similar rallies, protests and strikes in most of China's big cities.

Eventually, at the beginning of June, the government moved against the protesters; around 250,000 troops were deployed, some using live ammunition, and the death toll is estimated at around five hundred. Today, Chinese official policy is not to refer to the event but the world remembers the iconic photograph of an unarmed student facing a tank.

Today's poem is by Kabir, *The Time Before Death*:

> *Friend? Hope for the Guest while you are alive.*
> *Jump into experience while you are alive!*
> *Think ... and think ... while you are alive.*
> *What you call "salvation" belongs to the time*
> *before death*
> *If you don't break your ropes while you're alive,*
> *Do you think ghosts will do it after?*
> *The idea that the soul will join with the ecstatic*
> *just because the body is rotten –*
> *that is all fantasy.*
> *What is found now is found then.*
> *If you find nothing now,*
> *you will simply end up with an apartment in the*
> *City of Death.*
> *If you make love with the divine now, in the next*
> *life you will have the face of satisfied desire.*
> *So plunge into the truth, find out who the Teacher is,*
> *Believe in the Great Sound!*

Today I will reflect on being true to myself and living life as best I can.

April 20th

On this day in 1912 the writer and theatre manager Bram Stoker died. Stoker's career began as a journalist in Ireland. While writing theatre reviews in Dublin he became friendly with impresario and actor Henry Irving and moved to London to manage Irving's theatre, the Lyceum. He wrote his famous novel Dracula after meeting various people from Hungary. He never visited Transylvania.

Here is a suitably sinister piece of verse; it is from Shakespeare's evil-laden play, *Macbeth*:

> *Thrice the brinded cat hath mew'd.*
> *Thrice and once the hedge-pig whined.*
> *Harpier cries 'Tis time, 'tis time.*
> *Round about the cauldron go;*
> *In the poison'd entrails throw.*
> *Toad, that under cold stone*
> *Days and nights has thirty-one*
> *Swelter'd venom sleeping got,*
> *Boil thou first i' the charmed pot.*
> *Double, double toil and trouble;*
> *Fire burn, and cauldron bubble.*
> *Fillet of a fenny snake,*
> *In the cauldron boil and bake;*
> *Eye of newt and toe of frog,*
> *Wool of bat and tongue of dog,*
> *Adder's fork and blind-worm's sting,*
> *Lizard's leg and owlet's wing,*
> *For a charm of powerful trouble*
> *Like a hell-broth boil and bubble.*
> *Cool it with a baboon's blood,*
> *Then the charm is firm and good.*
> *By the pricking of my thumbs,*
> *Something wicked this way comes.*

Today I give thanks that I can cope with life's realities, a day at a time.

April 21st

On this day in 1926 Queen Elizabeth II was born in Mayfair, London. Her father had never expected to become monarch and nor did she. It was only in 1938, when her uncle Edward was famously 'pinched' by Mrs Simpson and abdicated, that everything changed for them. Today she is a worldwide icon of Britishness and a role model to millions.

In 1947, on her 21st birthday she made this pledge: "I declare before you all that my whole life, whether it be long or short, shall be devoted to your service and the service of our great imperial family to which we all belong." Probably nobody expected her to be still living by these principles well into the 21st century.

Here is Shakespeare's *Sonnet XXX*. Nobody knows to whom it was addressed, perhaps it was for Queen Elizabeth I:

> *When to the sessions of sweet silent thought*
> *I summon up remembrance of things past,*
> *I sigh the lack of many a thing I sought,*
> *And with old woes new wail my dear time's waste:*
> *Then can I drown an eye, unused to flow,*
> *For precious friends hid in death's dateless night,*
> *And weep afresh love's long since cancelled woe,*
> *And moan the expense of many a vanished sight:*
> *Then can I grieve at grievances foregone,*
> *And heavily from woe to woe tell o'er*
> *The sad account of fore-bemoanèd moan,*
> *Which I now pay as if not paid before.*
> *But if the while I think on thee, dear friend,*
> *All losses are restored and sorrows end.*

Today I will welcome the differences that make each one of us special.

April 22nd

On this day in 1899 the novelist Vladimir Nabokov was born. After an idyllic childhood in a leading St Petersburg family, Nabokov's world was upended by the Russian revolution in 1917. From then on the family moved through Europe, staying in Germany, Britain, Czechoslovakia and France, before fleeing to the USA when Hitler came to power.

Nabokov was brought up trilingual (Russian, French and English) and was a man of many interests – he liked chess, tennis, boxing and collecting butterflies. On the other hand he never learned to drive a car or live in a house of his own, and spent the last 16 years of his life living with his family at the Montreux Palace Hotel, Switzerland.

His work shows a fascination with words and language skills. He wrote books on butterflies and chess as well as novels. His most famous work is undoubtedly *Lolita*, the story of a grown man's highly unsuitable obsession with a 12 year old girl, which he made into a witty and entertaining narrative. It has been said that his pursuit of the girl is an allegory for his quest for a very rare butterfly.

Here is a poem by Heine, about a butterfly:

> The butterfly long loved the beautiful rose,
>   And flirted around all day;
>   While round him in turn with her golden caress,
>   Soft fluttered the sun's warm ray
> I know not with whom the rose was in love,
>   But I know that I loved them all.
>   The butterfly, rose, and the sun's bright ray,
>   The star and the bird's sweet call.

Today I will be grateful that I can identify with others; I will listen to their experiences and I will share my own.

April 23rd

On this day in 1564 the Spanish writer Miguel de Cervantes died, aged 69. Cervantes had been a soldier and sailor in his youth and had fought at the battle of Lepanto. Later his ship was taken by Barbary pirates and he spent five years in captivity before his family ransomed him.

He then worked for several years as a not very effective tax collector and naval agent before the success of *Don Quixote* gave him some financial security – he was 58 years old. This famous book shaped both the future of the modern novel and the Spanish language itself, which is often referred to as 'the language of Cervantes'.

Today's poem has to be the last few lines of Chesterton's *Lepanto*:

> *Don John pounding from the slaughter-painted poop,*
> *Purpling all the ocean like a bloody pirate's sloop,*
> *Scarlet running over on the silvers and the golds,*
> *Breaking of the hatches up and bursting of the holds,*
> *Thronging of the thousands up that labour under sea*
> *White for bliss and blind for sun and stunned for liberty.*
> *Vivat Hispania!*
> *Domino Gloria!*
> *Don John of Austria has set his people free!*
> *Cervantes on his galley sets the sword back in the sheath*
> *(Don John of Austria rides homeward with a wreath.)*
> *And he sees across a weary land a straggling road in Spain,*
> *Up which a lean and foolish knight forever rides in vain,*
> *And he smiles, but not as Sultans smile, and settles back the blade....*
> *(But Don John of Austria rides home from the Crusade.)*

Today I will accept that I do not have all the answers, but will trust that I have sufficient unto the day.

April 24th

On this day in 1815 the novelist Anthony Trollope was born. He drew on incidents in his own life when writing his famous series *Chronicles of Barsetshire*, such as debt, penury and corrupt electioneering.

He worked many years for the Post Office, and only retired following the success of his writing, in 1857. In his time he was one of the most successful novelists of the Victorian era and is still popular today.

Here is the last part of a poem by Rupert Brooke, which could have been about one of Trollope's imaginary villages, *The Old Village, Grantchester*:

> *Ah God! To see the branches stir*
> *Across the moon at Grantchester!*
> *To smell the thrilling-sweet and rotten*
> *Unforgettable, unforgotten*
> *River-smell, and hear the breeze*
> *Sobbing in the little trees. And after, ere the night is born,*
> *Do hares come out about the corn?*
> *Oh, is the water sweet and cool,*
> *Gentle and brown, above the pool?*
> *And laughs the immortal river still*
> *Under the mill, under the mill?*
> *Say, is there Beauty yet to find?*
> *And Certainty? And Quiet kind?*
> *Deep meadows yet, for to forget*
> *The lies, and truths, and pain? . . . oh! Yet*
> *Stands the Church clock at ten to three?*
> *And is there honey still for tea?*

Today I will find moments to be quiet and still, where I may listen to the voice of truth.

April 25th

On this day in 1873 the English poet and writer Walter de la Mare was born. He called himself Jack as he did not like his given name, Walter. He was the son of a Bank of England executive and until the age of 35 worked in an office.

He was very fond of children and wrote some beautiful stories for them. He was also drawn to mystery and magic, as his famous poem *The Listeners*, evokes so well.

De la Mare died aged 83 and his ashes are buried in St Paul's Cathedral, where he once sang as a choirboy. He must have read and been influenced by the Victorian purveyor of magic and romance, Christina Rossetti. Their styles can seem very similar.

Here is one of her poems, *Echo*:

> *Come to me in the silence of the night;*
> *Come in the speaking silence of a dream;*
> *Come with soft rounded cheeks and eyes as bright*
> *As sunlight on a stream;*
> *Come back in tears,*
> *O memory, hope, love of finished years.*
> *O dream how sweet, too sweet, too bitter sweet,*
> *Whose wakening should have been in Paradise,*
> *Where souls brimfull of love abide and meet;*
> *Where thirsting longing eyes*
> *Watch the slow door*
> *That opening, letting in, lets out no more.*
> *Yet come to me in dreams, that I may live*
> *My very life again though cold in death:*
> *Come back to me in dreams, that I may give*
> *Pulse for pulse, breath for breath:*
> *Speak low, lean low*
> *As long ago, my love, how long ago.*

Today I will avoid my old familiar lack of direction and instead ask for guidance, and listen when it is given.

April 26th

On this day in 1889 the Austrian and British philosopher Ludwig Wittgenstein was born in Vienna. As a child he went for a time to the same school as Adolf Hitler, though the two never met again afterwards. He fought for the Austrians in the First World War and was decorated for bravery.

He lived and studied at Cambridge for several years, though sometimes he would do menial jobs to unwind. His religious beliefs increased gradually and he inclined towards the Catholic religion. He died aged 62 and his last words were: 'tell them I have had a wonderful life'. For the man who famously said: 'I don't know why we are here, but I'm pretty sure that it is not in order to enjoy ourselves', that was quite a statement.

This poem, *The Human Abstract*, is by William Blake whose philosophy was simpler:

> Pity would be no more
> If we did not make somebody Poor;
> And Mercy no more could be
> If all were as happy as we.
> Then Cruelty knits a snare,
> And spreads his baits with care.
> Soon spreads the dismal shade
> Of Mystery over his head;
> And the Caterpillar and Fly
> Feed on the Mystery.
> And it bears the fruit of Deceit,
> Ruddy and sweet to eat;
> And the Raven his nest has made
> In its thickest shade.
> The Gods of the earth and sea
> Sought thro' Nature to find this Tree;
> But their search was all in vain:
> There grows one in the Human Brain.

Today I will share with others the problems I cannot resolve myself.

Apil 27th

On this day in 1737 the historian Edward Gibbon was born. He is chiefly remembered for his amazing *History of the Decline and Fall of the Roman Empire,* which set a high standard for history writing.

Some of his insights into the decline of great powers seem uncomfortably relevant today, such as: "The five marks of the Roman decaying culture: Concern with displaying affluence instead of building wealth; Obsession with sex and perversions of sex; Art becomes freakish and sensationalistic instead of creative and original; Widening disparity between very rich and very poor; Increased demand to live off the state."

This poem is by Thomas Macaulay from *Lays of Ancient Rome,* on the start of the Roman Empire:

> *Lars Porsena of Clusium*
> *By the Nine Gods he swore*
> *That the great house of Tarquin*
> *Should suffer wrong no more.*
> *By the Nine Gods he swore it,*
> *And named a trysting day,*
> *And bade his messengers ride forth,*
> *East and west and south and north,*
> *To summon his array.*
> *East and west and south and north*
> *The messengers ride fast,*
> *And tower and town and cottage*
> *Have heard the trumpet's blast.*
> *Shame on the false Etruscan*
> *Who lingers in his home,*
> *When Porsena of Clusium*
> *Is on the march for Rome.*

Today I will try to learn from the lessons of history.

April 28th

On this day in 1926 the American author Harper Lee was born. As a child, she lived in Monroeville, down the road from her friend Truman Capote. Her bestselling novel about racism and injustice in the Deep South, *To Kill a Mockingbird*, largely mirrored her own life – her father was a respected attorney who defended black people accused of murder and had failed to get an acquittal. It won her the Pulitzer Prize and the Presidential Medal of Freedom.

The book sold over ten million copies and she never wrote another one, saying she could not go through the emotional pain of publication again.

Here is a poem by Bengali poet Rabindranath Tagore, *Lost Star*:

*When the creation was new and all the stars shone in their first
Splendour, the gods held their assembly in the sky and sang
'Oh, the picture of perfection! The joy unalloyed!'
But one cried of a sudden
– 'It seems that somewhere there is a break in the chain of light
And one of the stars has been lost.'
The golden string of their harp snapped,
Their song stopped, and they cried in dismay
– 'Yes, that lost star was the best,
She was the glory of all heavens!'
From that day the search is unceasing for her,
And the cry goes on from one to the other
That in her the world has lost its one joy!
Only in the deepest silence of night the stars smile
And whisper among themselves
– 'Vain is this seeking! Unbroken perfection is over all!'*

Today I will remember the words of St. Peter: 'be ye all of one mind, having compassion one for another, not rendering evil for evil'.

April 29th

On this day in 1412 the French Saint and national heroine Joan of Arc was born at Domrémy, Eastern France. After convincing the king of her sincerity, she led the French army to spectacular victories against the English. But then she was captured and taken to Rouen, which was in English hands, and imprisoned.

She was tried on a charge of heresy and condemned to be burned at the stake. The trial was manifestly unjust and much of the argument concerned her cross-dressing, though she wore men's clothes and armour at certain times for two good reasons – to protect herself in battle and from rape in the camps (a very real danger). Joan did not use weapons in battle but carried a banner and was wounded several times.

She died bravely in the marketplace at Rouen holding a cross made for her by an English soldier. She was only 19. In two short years the Maid of Orleans had restored France's national pride, and 20 years after her death France won the 100 years war against England. A posthumous retrial in 1452, declared her innocent and a martyr. This is part of Joan's speech in Shakespeare's play *King Henry VI*:

> *Dauphin, I am by birth a shepherd's daughter,*
> *My wit untrain'd in any kind of art.*
> *Heaven and our Lady gracious hath it pleas'd*
> *To shine on my contemptible estate:*
> *Lo! Whilst I waited on my tender lambs,*
> *And to sun's parching heat display'd my cheeks,*
> *God's mother deigned to appear to me;*
> *And, in a vision full of majesty,*
> *Will'd me to leave my base vocation,*
> *And free my country from calamity.*

Today I reflect on those who overcame fear because they knew that they were doing right.

April 30th

On this day in 1945 Adolf Hitler committed suicide in his Berlin bunker. His Götterdämmerung (Twilight of the Gods) moment had been a while coming but had been foreseen by many after military defeats since 1942, failure on the Eastern front and the Normandy invasion in 1944. Hitler had angrily refused to accept defeat until the Red army were almost at the bunker doors. There had been several assassination attempts but none had succeeded.

Hitler married his mistress Eva Braun the day before and shot himself after she took a cyanide pill. Propaganda Minister Joseph Goebbels killed himself, his wife and their five young daughters at the same time. Many tyrants meet violent deaths; the assassins of Julius Caesar reportedly shouted 'sic semper tyrannis' (that's how it always is for tyrants). Some, perhaps regrettably, die in their beds. Joseph Stalin was one.

Perhaps one day a writer will come along to do it justice, as Shakespeare did for Macbeth:

> To-morrow, and to-morrow, and to-morrow,
> Creeps in this petty pace from day to day,
> To the last syllable of recorded time;
> And all our yesterdays have lighted fools
> The way to dusty death. Out, out, brief candle!
> Life's but a walking shadow, a poor player,
> That struts and frets his hour upon the stage,
> And then is heard no more. It is a tale
> Told by an idiot, full of sound and fury,
> Signifying nothing.

Today I will not let my inner peace be disturbed by the chaos around me.

May 1st

On this day in 1923 the American author Joseph Heller was born. Heller served in the US Air Force in the Second World War, an experience that he used in his memorable first novel, *Catch 22*.

He began to write the book by thinking up the first line: "It was love at first sight..." and it took him eight years to finish, but it was worth waiting for. Heller never repeated the success. Perhaps he struggled with inner demons.

Here is a poem, *Angels*, by Virginia Woolf, who knew a lot about inner demons:

> Five years after their rescue
> Of troops beaten back in Mons,
> She danced with them on the downs,
> Their forms like kites she reeled in
> With clouds, their haloes askew
> On waves of green escarpments
> Breaking into the sea. Beech-brown
> The combes she looked down upon
> While the angels held up her skirts,
> Rode the rhythms of her walking feet –
> Their wings no longer torn.
> In a host they balanced, on the alert
> For ancient armies in retreat
> Squatting in hunched hawthorns.
> One year after the armistice
> In the steep slopes of her temperament
> She kept them at her side, to banish
> The simpering angels of the house
> At whom, with the sedge, they would hiss.
> The angels of Mons were her guides

Today I will practice honesty and face up to my inner demons.

May 2nd

On this day in 1519 the Italian artist and polymath Leonardo da Vinci died. His biographer, Giorgio Vasari said: "In the normal course of events many men and women are born with remarkable talents; but occasionally, in a way that transcends nature, a single person is marvellously endowed by Heaven with beauty, grace and talent in such abundance that he leaves other men far behind."

There are thought to be only 15 extant paintings done by him, yet they are so exquisite that he is often held to be the greatest artist of all time.

Here is a poem by John Keats that Leonardo would have appreciated, *A Thing of Beauty*:

> A thing of beauty is a joy for ever:
> Its loveliness increases; it will never
> Pass into nothingness; but still will keep
> A bower quiet for us, and a sleep
> Full of sweet dreams, and health, and quiet breathing.
> Therefore, on every morrow, are we wreathing
> Some shape of beauty moves away the pall
> From our dark spirits. Such the sun, the moon,
> Trees old and young, sprouting a shady boon
> For simple sheep; and such are daffodils
> With the green world they live in; and clear rills
> That for themselves a cooling covert make
> 'Gainst the hot season; the mid-forest brake,
> Rich with a sprinkling of fair musk-rose blooms:
> And such too is the grandeur of the dooms
> We have imagined for the mighty dead;
> An endless fountain of immortal drink,
> Pouring unto us from the heaven's brink.

Today I am grateful for beautiful things, while remembering that I can find pleasure in the simple but beautiful things of life too.

May 3rd

On this day in 1469 the Italian writer and politician Niccolo Machiavelli was born in Florence. In the turbulent times of the Renaissance, as the various city states of Italy battled for influence, Machiavelli gained personal experience of the need for strong and decisive leadership.

His most famous work, *The Prince*, deals with good governance and was written after the Medici family had recovered power in the city. The book's apparent approval of devious and unscrupulous practices whereby the end justifies the means, by those in positions of government, has led to the use of the word 'Machiavellian'. It thus signifies a new approach whereby political realism is preferred to political idealism of the kind proposed by, for example, Plato in his *Republic*.

Here is a poem by William Butler Yeats, about life, *A Man Young And Old*:

Endure what life God gives and ask no longer span;
Cease to remember the delights of youth, travel-wearied aged man;
Delight becomes death-longing if all longing else be vain.
Even from that delight memory treasures so,
Death, despair, division of families, all entanglements of mankind
    grow,
As that old wandering beggar and these God-hated children know.
In the long echoing street the laughing dancers throng,
The bride is carried to the bridegroom's chamber through torchlight
    and tumultuous song;
I celebrate the silent kiss that ends short life or long.
Never to have lived is best, ancient writers say;
Never to have drawn the breath of life, never to have looked into
    the eye of day; the second best's a gay goodnight and quickly turn
    away.

Today I will set my own house in order and not seek to manipulate others.

May 4th

On this day in 1930 the Indian politician, lawyer and writer Mahatma Gandhi was imprisoned by the British. Gandhi was influenced by Plato and the American writer Thoreau in his use of passive resistance and non-violent protest to achieve political and humanitarian aims.

He was a very simple and honest man who had few possessions, lived mostly in communes and wore the Indian peasant garb. On showing up to meet King Edward VII dressed only in a loincloth, it was suggested he might have dressed more formally. His reply was: 'His Majesty was wearing enough for both of us'.

He was known and loved as the Father of India and his assassination by Hindu malcontents in 1948 was a huge shock. Over two million people attended his funeral. Bengali Poet Rabindranath Tagore knew Gandhi well.

Here is one of his poems, *Freedom*:

Freedom from fear is the freedom
I claim for you my motherland!
Freedom from the burden of the ages, bending your head,
Breaking your back, blinding your eyes to the beckoning
Call of the future;
Freedom from the shackles of slumber wherewith
You fasten yourself in night's stillness,
Mistrusting the star that speaks of truth's adventurous paths;
Freedom from the anarchy of destiny
Whole sails are weakly yielded to the blind uncertain winds,
And the helm to a hand ever rigid and cold as death.
Freedom from the insult of dwelling in a puppet's world,
Where movements are started through brainless wires,
Repeated through mindless habits,
Where figures wait with patience and obedience for the
Master of show, to be stirred into a mimicry of life.

Today I give thanks that I live free and I ask for help for those in prison.

May 5th

On this day in 1818 the political economist and philosopher Karl Marx was born in Germany. Reportedly a jovial companion and a loving husband and father, Marx's contribution to world Communism was ideological rather than practical.

Though championing the working class and actively promoting his ideas at meetings and in print, he is said to have played the stock market and never visited a factory.

He died in London in 1883, a stateless person and relatively unknown – 11 people attended the funeral. However his ideas were already spreading fast and may be said to have played a part in all of the great upheavals of the 20th century.

Marx wrote poetry too, some quite anarchic, here is the start of one entitled *Feelings*:

> *Never can I do in peace*
> *That with which my Soul's obsessed,*
> *Never take things at my ease;*
> *I must press on without rest.*
> *Others only know elation*
> *When things go their peaceful way,*
> *Free with self-congratulation,*
> *Giving thanks each time they pray.*
> *I am caught in endless strife,*
> *Endless ferment, endless dream;*
> *I cannot conform to Life,*
> *Will not travel with the stream.*
> *Heaven I would comprehend,*
> *I would draw the world to me;*
> *Loving, hating, I intend*
> *That my star shine brilliantly*

Today I ask for humility to accept the fact that I need help and the resolve to ask for it.

May 6th

On this day in 1861 the Bengali poet, artist and writer Rabindranath Tagore was born. His family were Brahmin landowners and Tagore spent time travelling when he was a child, a habit he continued for much of his life. Some of his schooling took place in England and he is said to have appreciated the English culture and regional folk songs.

He was a prolific writer, painter and musical composer and seems to have matched this with repeated travelling, visiting and lecturing in the United States, South America, Europe, the Middle East and Far East. In 1913 he became the first non-European to win the Nobel Prize for literature.

He was also knighted by the British but later renounced this in protest at a barbaric massacre. Tagore supported the Indian independence movement and at times worked with Gandhi, though they disagreed on some matters. His poetry has a dreamy and mystical style and has been widely translated from the original Bengali.

Here is one, *The Gardener*:

Who are you, reader, reading my poems an hundred years hence?
I cannot send you one single flower from this wealth of the spring,
*   one single streak of gold from yonder clouds.*
Open your doors and look abroad.
From your blossoming garden gather fragrant memories of the
*   vanished flowers of an hundred years before.*
In the joy of your heart may you feel the living joy that sang one
*   spring morning, sending its glad voice across an hundred years.*

Today I will remember that the more I give of myself the more I will be understood.

May 7th

On this day in 1812 the English poet Robert Browning was born. He was brought up by strict but loving parents and well educated – by the age of 12 he was writing verses.

His work was generally not well received until he came to public notice by marrying the poetess Elizabeth Barrett. He found the idea for his most famous poem, *The Pied Piper of Hamelin*, in his father's huge library. It tells of a mysterious piper who is hired to rid the town of a plague of rats but who, after being cheated of his payment for the task, lures away the town's children in revenge. Here is the start of it:

> *Hamelin Town's in Brunswick,*
> *By famous Hanover city;*
> *The river Weser, deep and wide,*
> *Washes its wall on the southern side;*
> *A pleasanter spot you never spied;*
> *But, when begins my ditty,*
> *Almost five hundred years ago,*
> *To see the townsfolk suffer so*
> *From vermin, was a pity.*
> *Rats!*
> *They fought the dogs and killed the cats,*
> *And bit the babies in the cradles,*
> *And ate the cheeses out of the vats,*
> *And licked the soup from the cooks' own ladles,*
> *Split open the kegs of salted sprats,*
> *Made nests inside men's Sunday hats,*
> *And even spoiled the women's chats,*
> *By drowning their speaking*
> *With shrieking and squeaking*
> *In fifty different sharps and flats.*

Today I will allow nothing to stop me from finding the good in my life and from putting it to best use.

May 8th

On this day in 1858 the English author and businessman John Meade Falkner was born. Apart from writing the much loved novel Moonfleet and several other stories and guidebooks, Falkner was remarkably, for six years during the First World War and after, chairman of Armstrong Whitworth, one of the world's largest war weapons manufacturers.

Moonfleet is an exciting story of smuggling and adventure on the Dorset Coast and was a school favourite for many years. Falkner based his imaginary village on real locations around Portland Bill. This is his poem called *After Trinity*:

> *We have done with dogma and divinity,*
> *Easter and Whitsun past,*
> *The long, long Sundays after Trinity,*
> *Are with us at last;*
> *The passionless Sundays after Trinity,*
> *Neither feast-day nor fast.*
> *Christmas comes with plenty,*
> *Lent spreads out its pall,*
> *But these are five and twenty,*
> *The longest Sundays of all;*
> *The placid Sundays after Trinity,*
> *Wheat-harvest, fruit-harvest, Fall.*
> *Spring with its burst is over,*
> *Summer has had its day,*
> *The scented grasses and clover*
> *Are cut, and dried into hay;*
> *The singing-birds are silent,*
> *And the swallows flown away.*
> *Twenty-fifth after Trinity,*
> *Kneel with the listening earth,*
> *Behind the Advent trumpets*
> *They are singing Emmanuel's birth.*

Today I will do my best and will stretch my potential to the fullest.

May 9th

On this day in 1265 the Italian poet Dante Alighieri was born in Florence. Dante's family were caught up in the fighting between various factions in the city at the time, and Dante himself fought in the battle of Campaldino between the Guelphs and the Ghibellines.

Because of the enmity going on in Florence, Dante was exiled in 1301 for the rest of his life and never returned to the city of his birth. During this exile he wrote his most famous work, the *Divine Comedy* (the word 'comedy' was used to describe a story that had a satisfactory ending). Dante is famous for his idea of courtly love which he experienced with his childhood fancy, Beatrice Portinari, which was never consummated. He wrote her several sonnets.

> *This one he wrote after meeting her for the last time:*
> *To every captive soul and gentle heart*
> *Into whose sight this present speech may come,*
> *So that they might write its meaning for me,*
> *Greetings, in their lord's name, who is Love.*
> *Already a third of the hours were almost past*
> *Of the time when all the stars were shining,*
> *When Love suddenly appeared to me*
> *Whose memory fills me with terror?*
> *Joyfully Love seemed to me to hold*
> *My heart in his hand, and held in his arms*
> *My lady wrapped in a cloth sleeping.*
> *Then he woke her, and that burning heart*
> *He fed to her reverently, she fearing,*
> *Afterwards he went not to be seen weeping.*

Today I will remember the words of Kahlil Gibran: "there are those who have little and give it all. These are the believers in life and the bounty of life and their coffers are never empty". I cannot receive until I give.

May 10th

On this day in 1915 the English writer Monica Dickens was born. The unconventional daughter of a well-to-do family, and a great granddaughter of Charles Dickens, on leaving school she chose to go into service as a housemaid and cook.

This led to her writing her first book about her experiences, *One Pair of Hands* which was an instant success and has never been out of print. She worked throughout the Second World War and wrote books about her various jobs, and later moved to the United States after marrying an American.

She lived there happily for over 30 years, with two adopted daughters, still writing stories about England. During this time she was instrumental in starting the Samaritans movement in the US through her friendship with founder Dr Chad Varah. She returned to England after her husband's death and continued to write and support good causes.

Here is a poem by American James Weldon Johnson, whose cause was American civil rights, something that Monica Dickens would have recognised, *I Hear the Stars Still Singing*:

> I hear the stars still singing
> To the beautiful, silent night,
> As they speed with noiseless winging
> Their ever westward flight.
> I hear the waves still falling
> On the stretch of lonely shore,
> But the sound of a sweet voice calling
> I shall hear, alas! no more

Today I will examine my relationships and work to improve them wherever possible.

May 11th

On this day in 1904 the Spanish painter Salvador Dali was born. Dali's work was matched by his extraordinary behaviour. As befitted a surrealist, his publicity stunts were highly unusual, such as giving a lecture in a diving suit and travelling with a pet ocelot. He was a great friend of Federico Garcia Lorca.

Here is part of Lorca's poem *Ode to Salvador Dali*:

Oh Salvador Dali, of the olive-colored voice!
I speak of what your person and your paintings tell me.
I do not praise your halting adolescent brush,
but I sing the steady aim of your arrows.
I sing your fair struggle of Catalan lights,
your love of what might be made clear.
I sing your astronomical and tender heart,
a never-wounded deck of French cards.
I sing your restless longing for the statue,
your fear of the feelings that await you in the street.
I sing the small sea siren who sings to you,
riding her bicycle of corals and conches.
But above all I sing a common thought
that joins us in the dark and golden hours.
The light that blinds our eyes is not art.
Rather it is love, friendship, crossed swords.
May fingerprints of blood on gold
streak the heart of eternal Catalunya.
May stars like falconless fists shine on you,
while your painting and your life break into flower.
Don't watch the water clock with its membraned wings
or the hard scythe of the allegory.
Always in the air, dress and undress your brush
before the sea peopled with sailors and ships

Today I will do something that helps me recognise that I am a good person who should feel love for himself.

May 12th

On this day in 1820 the English nurse and administrator Florence Nightingale was born in Florence, Italy. She worked as a nurse in London and was sent with a small party of volunteers to Scutari (part of Istanbul) where the main hospital for the wounded from the Crimean War was located.

By imposing basic standards of sanitation and nutrition she was able to vastly improve the conditions. By the time she returned from the Crimea, the 'Lady with the Lamp' was famous and a potent force for change.

She never married and seemingly put her vocation first. Her most persistent suitor was the poet Richard Monckton Milnes Houghton, who courted her for nine years, only to be rejected.

His poem *Shadows*, probably refers to the doomed affair:

> They seem'd, to those who saw them meet,
> The casual friends of every day;
> Her smile was undisturb'd and sweet,
> His courtesy was free and gay.
> But yet if one the other's name
> In some unguarded moment heard,
> The heart you thought so calm and tame
> Would struggle like a captured bird
> And letters of mere formal phrase
> Were blister'd with repeated tears,
> And this was not the work of days,
> But had gone on for years and years!
> Alas, that love was not too strong
> For maiden shame and manly pride!
> Alas, that they delay'd so long
> The goal of mutual bliss beside!

Today I will try to be steadfast in all that I set out to do.

May 13th

On this day in 1907 the English novelist Daphne Du Maurier was born. Her books *Rebecca* and *Jamaica Inn* still remain among the nation's best loved works. Du Maurier came from an artistic family and seems to have been a very private person.

Although happily married with three children, her letters and memoirs found after her death revealed a passionate and bisexual secret life. Daphne Du Maurier was a feisty woman and a passionate admirer of the Brontës.

Here is part of Emily Brontë's famous poem, *No Coward Soul Is Mine*:

> No coward soul is mine
> No trembler in the world's storm-troubled sphere
> I see Heaven's glories shine
> And Faith shines equal arming me from Fear
> O God within my breast
> Almighty ever-present Deity
> Life, that in me hast rest,
> As I Undying Life, have power in Thee
> Vain are the thousand creeds
> That move men's hearts, unutterably vain,
> Worthless as withered weeds
> Or idlest froth amid the boundless main
> To waken doubt in one
> Holding so fast by thy infinity,
> So surely anchored on
> The steadfast rock of Immortality.
> There is not room for Death
> Nor atom that his might could render void
> Since thou art Being and Breath
> And what thou art may never be destroyed.

Today I will remember that self-improvement is about seeking progress rather than perfection.

May 14th

On this day in 1925 the novel *Mrs Dalloway* by Virginia Woolf was published. The action takes place in the course of a single June day and is in the form of a 'stream of consciousness'. As such it is seen as a response to James Joyce's *Ulysses*, first published three years earlier.

Virginia and her husband Leonard had to turn down the chance for their Hogarth Press to publish *Ulysses* in 1919, because of England's obscenity laws. Her own book addresses subjects that were uncomfortable at the time, such as mental illness, suicide, regret over choice of husband, and lesbianism. Much of this mirrored Woolf's own life, including mental breakdown, before her own suicide in 1941.

This poem by Elizabeth Barrett Browning describes a similar mental turmoil, *Chorus of Eden Spirits*:

> *Hearken, oh hearken! Let your souls behind you*
> *Turn, gently moved!*
> *Our voices feel along the Dread to find you,*
> *O lost, beloved!*
> *Through the thick-shielded and strong-marshalled angels,*
> *They press and pierce:*
> *Our requiems follow fast on our evangels, –*
> *Voice throbs in verse.*
> *We are but orphaned spirits left in Eden*
> *A time ago:*
> *God gave us golden cups, and we were bidden*
> *To feed you so.*
> *And when upon you, weary after roaming,*
> *Death's seal is put,*
> *By the foregone ye shall discern the coming,*
> *Through eyelids shut.*

Today I ask for the serenity to accept the things I cannot change.

May 15th

On this day in 1659 the English aristocrat, socialite, writer and poet Lady Mary Wortley Montague was born. An independent and strong minded woman, she spent several years in Constantinople where her husband was ambassador and later, after they separated, travelled and lived extensively in Europe. Her letters from Turkey contain descriptions of a Turkish bath and the horror of Turkish women who saw her corsets as instruments of torture.

Here is part of a poem written to her by Alexander Pope, an admirer:

In beauty, or wit, no mortal as yet
To question your empire has dared:
But men of discerning
Have thought that in learning
To yield to a lady was hard.
'T was a woman at first
(Indeed she was curst)
In knowledge that tasted delight,
Then bravely, fair dame,
Resume the old claim,
Which to your whole sex does belong;
And let men receive,
From a second bright Eve,
The knowledge of right and of wrong.
But if the first Eve
Hard doom did receive,
When only one apple had she,
What a punishment new
Shall be found out for you,
Who tasting, have robb'd the whole tree?

Today I will reflect upon change and the need sometimes to challenge conventions.

May 16th

On this day in 1763 in London, Dr Samuel Johnson met his future biographer, James Boswell, for the first time. It was not love at first sight. Boswell tried unsuccessfully to hide the fact that he was a Scot but when it came out he said: "Indeed I come from Scotland but I cannot help it."

To which Johnson replied: "That I find is what a very great many of your countrymen cannot help." However they soon met again and became good friends. Somehow the brash young Boswell was the perfect foil for the weighty old man.

Boswell wrote after that first meeting: "a Man of a most dreadful appearance. He is very slovenly in his dress and speaks with a most uncouth voice. Yet his great knowledge, and strength of expression command vast respect and render him excellent company."

The socially ambitious Boswell is only known to have written one (not very good) poem entitled *The Cub at Newmarket*. Typically, he dedicated it to the Prince of Wales, without his permission. His prose is much better:

> *Poets, for most part, have been poor;*
> *Experience tells us; Proof too sure.*
> *"Ay, may be so," Lord Rich exclaims,*
> *Who Fortune's Will incessant blames,*
> *"It may be so; but yet, confound 'em,*
> *"They still have Jollity around 'em."*
> *Pray, my good Lord, 'tis no Offence*
> *To ask by rules of common sense,*
> *Is not this distribution right?*
> *At least I view it in that light;*
> *For 'tis but just that ev'ry Creature*
> *Should have some favour from Dame Nature.*

Today I will remember that if I can love others without expecting to be loved back, I will most likely receive love in return.

May 17th

On this day in 1510 the Italian painter Sandro Botticelli died. Very little detail is known about his life: he was apprenticed to Friar Filippo Lippi, was greatly influenced by the puritanical monk Savonarola to the extent of burning several of his paintings in the famous 'bonfire of the vanities' and seems to have harboured an unrequited love for a married lady named Simonetta Vespucci, though other commentators have hinted that he might have been homosexual.

None of this particularly matters when one contemplates his paintings which, to most people, represent some of the most beautiful figurative works of art ever produced.

Here is a beautiful poem, *There's a Moon Inside my Body* by the mystic poet Kabir who lived in India, around the same time as Botticelli:

> *The moon shines in my body, but my blind eyes cannot see it:*
> *The moon is within me, and so is the sun.*
> *The unstruck drum of Eternity is sounded within me; but my deaf*
> * ears cannot hear it.*
> *So long as man clamours for the I and the Mine, his works are as*
> * naught:*
> *When all love of the I and the Mine is dead, then the work of the*
> * Lord is done.*
> *For work has no other aim than the getting of knowledge:*
> *When that comes, then work is put away.*
> *The flower blooms for the fruit: when the fruit comes, the flower*
> * withers.*
> *The musk is in the deer, but it seeks it not within itself: it wanders in*
> * quest of grass.*

Today I will keep it simple and be grateful for the beauty around me.

May 18th

On this day in 1872 the English philosopher and Nobel Prize winner Bertrand Russell was born. He won the Nobel Prize for literature after publishing his *Principia Mathematica* and other works but is today equally admired for his fearless political campaigning for peace and nuclear disarmament.

He was arrested many times at demonstrations and received a seven day jail sentence for breach of the peace at the age of 89. Russell received many honours including the OBE from King George VI who, mindful of his political activities, said: "You have sometimes behaved in a manner that would not do if generally adopted". Russell later claimed that he nearly replied: "That's right, just like your brother" (who abandoned the throne for his mistress, Mrs Simpson).

I think he would have liked this poem by George William Russell (no relation), *Brotherhood*:

Twilight, a blossom grey in shadowy valleys dwells:
Under the radiant dark the deep blue-tinted bells
In quietness re-image heaven within their blooms,
Sapphire and gold and mystery. What strange perfumes,
Out of what deeps arising, all the flower-bells fling,
Unknowing the enchanted odorous song they sing!
Oh, never was an eve so living yet: the wood
Stirs not but breathes enraptured quietude.
Here in these shades the ancient knows itself, the soul,
And out of slumber waking starts unto the goal.
What bright companions nod and go along with it!
Out of the teeming dark what dusky creatures flit,
That through the long leagues of the island night above
Come by me, wandering, whispering, beseeching love;
As in the twilight children gather close and press
Nigh and more nigh with shadowy tenderness

Today I will take time to recognise my talents with gratitude.

May 19th

On this day in 1925 the African – American rights activist Malcolm X was born. His family name was Little, but he called himself Malcolm X to symbolise the loss of his true African name when his forbears were taken into slavery. He converted to Islam and joined the Nation of Islam movement that advocated segregation and violence to achieve their goals.

He became disenchanted and left to join the moderate Sufi sect. However his acrimonious falling out with the Nation of Islam (who viewed him as a traitor) caused strong feelings. In 1965, he was assassinated by three members of the movement. Today he is seen as a great leader in the struggle for racial equality, a man whose methods were not always right but whose intentions were generally good. This poem, by AE Housman, *Be Still my Soul* about an unquiet soul, could refer to him:

> Be still, my soul, be still; the arms you bear are brittle,
> Earth and high heaven are fixt of old and founded stron
> Think rather, – call to thought, if now you grieve a little,
> The days when we had rest, O soul, for they were long.
> Men loved unkindness then, but lightless in the quarry
> I slept and saw not; tears fell down, I did not mourn;
> Sweat ran and blood sprang out and I was never sorry:
> Then it was well with me, in days ere I was born.
> Now, and I muse for why and never find the reason,
> I pace the earth, and drink the air, and feel the sun.
> Be still, be still, my soul; it is but for a season:
> Let us endure an hour and see injustice done.
> Ay, look: high heaven and earth ail from the prime foundation
> All thoughts to rive the heart are here, and all are vain:
> Horror and scorn and hate and fear and indignation –
> Oh why did I awake? When shall I sleep again?

Today I will remember that all men are created equal.

May 20th

On this day in 1609 Shakespeare's sonnets were first published in London. Shakespeare's writings are well known for their many hidden meanings and illusions. The sonnets have baffled commentators for centuries. We will probably never know to whom they were addressed, just as we don't really know who the true Shakespeare was, the man behind the facade.

We cannot even be sure what his sexual preferences were and reading the sonnets for clues just results in more confusion. It is tempting to speculate that, given his inventiveness, he might have left a clue that would unlock the truth somewhere in his writings. It is as if Shakespeare is standing in the shadows gently mocking us. And so it is likely to remain. Our best choice is simply to enjoy the beauty of the poetry.

Here is one that many consider the most beautiful sonnet of all, *Sonnet XVIII* – was it written to a man or a woman? Shall I compare thee to a summer's day?

Thou art more lovely and more temperate:
Rough winds do shake the darling buds of May,
And summer's lease hath all too short a date;
Sometime too hot the eye of heaven shines,
And often is his gold complexion dimm'd;
And every fair from fair sometime declines,
By chance or nature's changing course untrimm'd;
But thy eternal summer shall not fade,
Nor lose possession of that fair thou ow'st;
Nor shall death brag thou wander'st in his shade,
When in eternal lines to time thou grow'st:
    So long as men can breathe or eyes can see,
    So long lives this, and this gives life to thee.

Today I will remember to be grateful for what I know and have.

May 21st

On this day in 1688 the English poet Alexander Pope was born. He grew up extremely well educated, mostly through his own efforts, and made a career as a writer and poet from an early age. He suffered from bone disease and grew to only 4 feet 6 inches tall. Nevertheless he was very sociable and knew many of the literary figures of the day.

He formed the Scriblerus Club that focused on the writing of satire, and became a popular London figure. As well as translating Homer's great works, the *Iliad* and the *Odyssey*, he wrote several long narrative poem in the classical style, the best known being the *Rape of the Lock*. Pope lived in Twickenham, West London, where his house with its famous Grotto was often full of visitors.

Here is a poem by his friend, Lady Mary Wortley Montague – perhaps it was written in Pope's garden, *Hymn to the Moon*:

> Thou silver deity of secret night,
>   Direct my footsteps through the woodland shade;
> Thou conscious witness of unknown delight,
>   The Lover's guardian, and the Muse's aid!
> By thy pale beams I solitary rove,
>   To thee my tender grief confide;
> Serenely sweet you gild the silent grove,
>   My friend, my goddess, and my guide.
> E'en thee, fair queen, from thy amazing height,
>   The charms of young Endymion drew;
> Veil'd with the mantle of concealing night;
>   With all thy greatness and thy coldness too.

Today I will remember the words of Epictetus: "so you too moderate your desires, that they are not too much."

May 22nd

On this day in 1859 the English author Sir Arthur Conan Doyle was born. Famous as the creator of Sherlock Holmes, he was a physician and ophthalmologist whose business was not successful – he started writing stories while waiting for clients to turn up. Luckily for us, not many did.

Conan Doyle eventually got fed up with Holmes and his sidekick Dr Watson and killed them both off, hoping to concentrate on more serious historical writing. However, the public outcry was such that he was forced to resurrect them. He also wrote poetry, some of it with a mysterious and ominous feel, not unlike his books.

Here is one, *A Tragedy*:

> *Who's that walking on the moorland?*
> *Who's that moving on the hill?*
> *They are passing 'mid the bracken,*
> *But the shadows grow and blacken*
> *And I cannot see them clearly on the hill.*
> *Who's that calling on the moorland?*
> *Who's that crying on the hill?*
> *Was it bird or was it human,*
> *Was it child, or man, or woman,*
> *Who was calling so sadly on the hill?*
> *Who's that running on the moorland?*
> *Who's that flying on the hill?*
> *He is there – and there again,*
> *But you cannot see him plain,*
> *For the shadow lies so darkly on the hill.*
> *What's that lying in the heather?*
> *What's that lurking on the hill?*
> *My horse will go no nearer,*
> *And I cannot see it clearer,*
> *But there's something that is lying on the hill.*

Today I will not make idle moments an excuse to do nothing.

May 23rd

On this day in 1936 the American psychiatrist and writer M Scott Peck was born. His best-selling book, *The Road Less Travelled*, with its unusual views on feelings and behaviours, has led thousands to reconsider their position in life. His perspective on love for example, as not a feeling, but an activity and an investment, caused many to revisit their most powerful motivation.

He defines love as "the will to extend one's self for the purpose of nurturing one's own or another's spiritual growth". Less well known is that Peck was also an exorcist who helped many people suffering from demonic possession. His book *Glimpses of the Devil* is a factual and often chilling account of several exorcisms undertaken in the New York area.

Today's poem is about playwright Christopher Marlowe's *Dr Faustus*, a man who sold himself to the devil for short term gain. These are the famous lines spoken by Faustus as time runs out for him and the devil comes to claim him:

> *Ah Faustus, now hast thou but one bare hour to live,*
> *And then thou must be damned perpetually!*
> *Stand still you ever-moving spheres of Heaven,*
> *That time may cease and midnight never come;*
> *Fair Nature's eye, rise, rise again and make*
> *Perpetual day; or let this hour be but*
> *A year, a month, a week, a natural day,*
> *That Faustus may repent and save his soul!*
> *O lente, lente, currite noctis equi.*
> *The stars move still, time runs the clock will strike,*
> *The Devil will come and Faustus must be damned.*

Today I ask to make the right choices, between short term gain and long term benefit. I will not sell my soul to the devil.

May 24th

On this day in 1950 British Field Marshall Archibald Percival Wavell died. Wavell was a well-known general in the Second World War where he came up against Rommel in North Africa. Between 1943 and 1947 he was appointed Viceroy of India, shortly before the granting of independence.

He was an upright, cultured and sensitive man, judged by some to be too kind to be a great commander. On retirement, he produced the much loved anthology of poetry, *Other Men's Flowers*. In this he added his own pithy remarks and even one of his own poems.

This poem from *Other Men's Flowers*, is by John Dryden, *Alexander's Feast*:

'Twas at the royal feast for Persia won
By Philip's warlike son –
Aloft in awful state
The godlike hero sate
On his imperial throne;
His valiant peers were placed around,
Their brows with roses and with myrtles bound
(So should desert in arms be crown'd);
The lovely Thais by his side
Sate like a blooming Eastern bride
In flower of youth and beauty's pride: –
Happy, happy, happy pair!
None but the brave
None but the brave
None but the brave deserves the fair!

Today I seek self-honesty; to be able to say when I am wrong and to make amends when it is right to do so.

May 25th

O n this day in 1803 the American writer and poet Ralph Waldo Emerson was born. Known today as a leader of the Romantic Movement, he wrote the well-known *Concord Hymn* that features on the Concord monument.

It begins:

> *By the rude bridge that arched the flood,*
> *Their flag to April's breeze unfurled,*
> *Here once the embattled farmers stood,*
> *And fired the shot heard round the world.*

Although he was ordained as a pastor, Emerson eschewed organised religion in favour of transcendentalism, a movement that he was instrumental in starting. Here is his strange but magical poem, *Brahma:*

> *If the red slayer think he slays,*
> *Or if the slain think he is slain,*
> *They know not well the subtle ways*
> *I keep, and pass, and turn again.*
> *Far or forgot to me is near;*
> *Shadow and sunlight are the same;*
> *The vanished gods to me appear;*
> *And one to me are shame and fame.*
> *They reckon ill who leave me out;*
> *When me they fly, I am the wings;*
> *I am the doubter and the doubt,*
> *And I the hymn the Brahmin sings.*
> *The strong gods pine for my abode,*
> *And pine in vain the sacred Seven;*
> *But thou, meek lover of the good!*
> *Find me, and turn thy back on heaven.*

Today I will remember that the truth is not always readily apparent but can be found with perseverance.

May 26th

On this day in 1859 the English poet Alfred Edward (AE) Housman was born. He is best remembered today for his lyrical and evocative poetry especially that set in Shropshire where he grew up. His collection of poems entitled *A Shropshire Lad* is especially well known.

Housman always considered his poetry second to his academic work – he was a Professor of Latin at Cambridge. Throughout his life he struggled with feelings for other men and was sympathetic towards the difficulties of Oscar Wilde. Much of his poetry relates to a golden age in the countryside, before the First World War.

Here is his poem, *On Wenlock Edge*:

> *On Wenlock Edge the wood's in trouble;*
> *His forest fleece the Wrekin heaves;*
> *The gale, it plies the saplings double,*
> *And thick on Severn snow the leaves.*
> *'Twould blow like this through holt and hanger*
> *When Uricon the city stood:*
> *'Tis the old wind in the old anger,*
> *But then it threshed another wood.*
> *Then, 'twas before my time, the Roman*
> *At yonder heaving hill would stare:*
> *The blood that warms an English yeoman,*
> *The thoughts that hurt him, they were there.*
> *There, like the wind through woods in riot,*
> *Through him the gale of life blew high;*
> *The tree of man was never quiet:*
> *Then 'twas the Roman, now 'tis I.*
> *The gale, it plies the saplings double,*
> *It blows so hard, 'twill soon be gone:*
> *To-day the Roman and his trouble*
> *Are ashes under Uricon.*

Today I accept responsibility for myself and my life.

May 27th

On this day in 1703 in Russia, the Tsar Peter the Great founded the northern city of St Petersburg. It was to become Russia's capital city for two centuries. Peter had spent several months touring the great cities of Europe, including London, and recruited many leading architects and engineers during his travels.

An army of serfs was conscripted for the construction labour. Work conditions were often terrible, especially in winter, and thousands died. As early as 1712 it had become the seat of government. Today it is Russia's second city and its vast baroque and neo-classical buildings and vibrant cultural life make it a popular tourist destination.

Here is a poem by CP Cavafy called *The City* which says that we carry our problems within us:

> You said: "I'll go to another country, go to another shore,
> find another city better than this one.
> Whatever I try to do is fated to turn out wrong
> and my heart lies buried like something dead.
> How long can I let my mind moulder in this place?
> Wherever I turn, wherever I look,
> I see the black ruins of my life, here,
> where I've spent so many years, wasted them, destroyed them
>   totally."
> You won't find a new country, won't find another shore.
> This city will always pursue you.
> You'll walk the same streets, grow old
> in the same neighborhoods, turn gray in these same houses.
> You'll always end up in this city. Don't hope for things elsewhere:
> there's no ship for you, there's no road.
> Now that you've wasted your life here, in this small corner,
> you've destroyed it everywhere in the world.

Today I will take responsibility for my problems and not seek to run away.

May 28th

On this day in 1140 the Chinese poet, statesman and military leader Xin Qiji (pronounced 'Shin Chee Gee") was born. His life seems to have been one of service to the Han emperors through fighting to rid the North of China from the Jin rulers, a nomadic people regarded as barbarians.

Though a successful commander, Xin Qiji was not appreciated by the emperors until he was too old to be of much use. His poetry is a mixture of beautiful imagery and wistfulness:

> *I wrote this for fun when drunk.*
> *A thousand hands held high to heaven*
> *Swept along with a torrent of shouts*
> *A gold seal hanging from my belt*
> *Big as a ladle*
> *Our riders came in swarms with bows and swords*
> *I commanded them to quickly cover front and rear*
> *We tried all kinds of subterfuge*
> *Like children fighting in the grass*
> *Determined to prevail futility!*
> *Forget the furrow in my brow*
> *With hair turned white*
> *It's useless to look back*
> *Idle now, I pass the time of day*
> *With mountain friends*
> *See those sheep and cattle on the hillside,*
> *Who could sort the smart from stupid?*
> *I've taken to tending plants and willows*
> *Dreading visitors*
> *Tell them I'm drunk this morning*

Today I ask that I will do my best, not so as to please others but so as to give myself respect.

May 29th

On this day in 1874 the English writer Gilbert Keith (GK) Chesterton was born. A prolific writer of lay theology and philosophy as well as novels and poetry, he wrote with wit and humour about serious subjects such a morality and Christian beliefs.

Here he criticises his contemporary Oscar Wilde's attitude of 'taking your pleasures where you can find them': "The carpe diem religion is not the religion of happy people, but of very unhappy people. Great joy does not gather the rosebuds while it may; its eyes are fixed on the immortal rose which Dante saw." Chesterton was much loved and admired by his contemporaries.

Here is one of his typical poems that combines light-heartedness with a serious message, *The Donkey*:

> When fishes flew and forests walked
>   And figs grew upon thorn,
> Some moment when the moon was blood
>   Then surely I was born.
> With monstrous head and sickening cry
>   And ears like errant wings,
> The devil's walking parody
>   On all four-footed things.
> The tattered outlaw of the earth,
>   Of ancient crooked will;
> Starve, scourge, deride me: I am dumb,
>   I keep my secret still.
> Fools! For I also had my hour;
>   One far fierce hour and sweet:
> There was a shout about my ears,
>   And palms before my feet.

Today I will remember the words of John Milton: They also serve who only stand and wait (Sonnet on His Blindness).

May 30th

On this day in 1593 the English playwright Christopher Marlowe was stabbed to death in a London pub. Although he was born in 1564, the same year as Shakespeare, Marlowe's life was short.

As with Shakespeare, little detail is known. He was certainly well educated, went to Cambridge University and was a big influence on Shakespeare. Marlowe may have worked as a spy for the government. Some commentators even suggest that he faked his death and continued working under the nom de plume of 'William Shakespeare'.

The report of the inquest does not make things clear. It seems that Marlowe had spent all day in a lodging house in Deptford, with three men: all three had been employees of Robert Walsingham, Queen Elizabeth's minister, which raises several questions. They argued over a 'reckoning', possibly the bill for their food and drink, and words turned to blows. Marlowe was stabbed above the eye and died instantly. We can only speculate as to the truth. Certainly Marlowe wrote some beautiful poetry.

Here is an extract, from his play *The Jew of Malta*:

> But we will leave this paltry land,
> And sail from hence to Greece, to lovely Greece;
> I'll be thy Jason, thou my golden fleece;
> Where painted carpets o'er the meads are hurl'd,
> And Bacchus' vineyards overspread the world,
> Where woods and forests go in goodly green,
> I'll be Adonis, thou shalt be Love's Queen;
> The meads, the orchards, and the primrose-lanes,
> Instead of sedge and reed, bear sugar-canes:
> Thou in those groves, by Dis above,
> Shalt live with me, and be my love.

Today I will ask for the courage and guidance that I need to help me achieve my goals.

May 31st

On this day in 1279 BC, Rameses II of Egypt became Pharaoh. Said by many to be the greatest of all the pharaohs, this warrior king won many battles and extended Egypt's power and influence throughout the Middle East – a thousand years before the Roman Empire began to emerge. Rameses died aged about 90.

His mummy has survived and was subject to forensic examination in Paris. He is also known as Ozymandias and many temples and monuments were built in his name, including the one that inspired Shelley to write his most famous poem: *Ozymandias*. Shelley was travelling with his friend and fellow poet Horace Smith at the time and they each wrote a poem on the subject.

Here is Horace's effort, also called *Ozymandias*:

> In Egypt's sandy silence, all alone,
> Stands a gigantic Leg, which far off throws
> The only shadow that the Desert knows:
> "I am great Ozymandias," saith the stone,
> "The King of Kings; this mighty City shows
> "The wonders of my hand." The City's gone,
> Nought but the Leg remaining to disclose
> The site of this forgotten Babylon.
> We wonder, and some Hunter may express
> Wonder like ours, when thro' the wilderness
> Where London stood, holding the Wolf in chace,
> He meets some fragment huge, and stops to guess
> What powerful but unrecorded race
> Once dwelt in that annihilated place.

Today I will remember Christ's words from the Sermon on the Mount – Blessed are the meek, for they shall inherit the earth.

June 1st

On this day in 1971 the American pastor, academic and theologian Reinhold Niebuhr died. Born into a devout German immigrant family, Niebuhr worked in Detroit for many years and was outspoken in his support of workers' rights as well as against Nazism, McCarthyism and racism.

His writings have been influential on many well-known public figures including US presidents Carter and Obama; Martin Luther King and Hillary Clinton. Niebuhr is also famous as the composer of the Serenity Prayer: "God grant me the serenity to accept the things I cannot change, courage to change the things I can and the wisdom to know the difference".

This prayer, conceived in 1937, is especially beloved by self-help fellowships in the fight against addiction, such as Alcoholics Anonymous. It is also a source of comfort and calm to anyone suffering stress or anxiety.

As such it is not unlike the prayer of St Francis:

> *Lord, make me an instrument of Your peace;*
> *Where there is hatred, let me sow love;*
> *Where there is injury, pardon;*
> *Where there is discord, harmony;*
> *Where there is error, truth;*
> *Where there is doubt, faith;*
> *Where there is despair, hope;*
> *Where there is darkness, light;*
> *And where there is sadness, joy.*
> *O Divine Master, Grant that I may not so much seek*
> *To be consoled as to console;*
> *To be understood as to understand;*
> *To be loved as to love.*
> *For it is in giving that we receive;*
> *It is in pardoning that we are pardoned;*
> *And it is in dying that we are born to eternal life.*

Today I shall say the Serenity Prayer, as I do every day.

June 2nd

On this day in 1840 the English author and poet Thomas Hardy was born. Hardy qualified as an architect but practised this profession very little. He is known for his romantic yet realistic portrayals of country life and his novels; *Far From the Madding Crowd*, *Tess of the D'Urbervilles* and *Under the Greenwood Tree* are still popular.

Hardy struggled for much of his career with Victorian conservative values and several of his books received a bad press because of their sympathetic treatment of fallen women. His novel *Jude the Obscure* was sometimes sold in paper bags because of its treatment of sex and religion.

Here is one of his poems, *Places*:

> *Nobody says: Ah, that is the place*
> *Where chanced, in the hollow of years ago,*
> *What none of the Three Towns cared to know –*
> *The birth of a little girl of grace*
> *The sweetest the house saw, first or last;*
> *Yet it was so on that day long past.*
> *Night, morn, and noon.*
> *Nobody calls to mind that here*
> *Upon Boterel Hill, where the carters skid,*
> *With cheeks whose airy flush outbid*
> *Fresh fruit in bloom, and free of fear,*
> *She cantered down, as if she must fall*
> *(Though she never did),*
> *To the charm of all.*
> *Nay: one there is to whom these things,*
> *That nobody else's mind calls back,*
> *Have a savour that scenes in being lack,*
> *And a presence more than the actual brings;*
> *To whom to-day is beneaped and stale,*
> *And its urgent clack but a vapid tale*

Today I will try not to judge, but to understand and to help.

June 3rd

On this day in 1924 the Czech author Franz Kafka died. Anyone who reads his work is likely to be horrified and strangely, amused. Here is the opening of his famous story *The Metamorphosis*: "As Gregor Samsa awoke one morning from uneasy dreams he found himself transformed in his bed into a gigantic insect."

It is horrific but what comes across from reading the story is the inner strength that Gregor finds in dealing with his terrible dilemma, in the face of alienation from his family and the world and, ultimately, himself. This poem *The Show*, by Wilfred Owen has some of the horror found in Kafka's prose:

> My soul looked down from a vague height with Death,
> As unremembering how I rose or why,
> And saw a sad land, weak with sweats of dearth,
> Gray, cratered like the moon with hollow woe,
> And fitted with great pocks and scabs of plaques.
> Across its beard, that horror of harsh wire,
> There moved thin caterpillars, slowly uncoiled.
> It seemed they pushed themselves to be as plugs
> Of ditches, where they writhed and shrivelled, killed.
> By them had slimy paths been trailed and scraped
> Round myriad warts that might be little hills.
> On dithering feet upgathered, more and more,
> Brown strings towards strings of gray, with bristling spines,
> All migrants from green fields, intent on mire.
> Those that were gray, of more abundant spawns,
> Ramped on the rest and ate them and were eaten.
> I saw their bitten backs curve, loop, and straighten,
> I watched those agonies curl, lift, and flatten.
> Whereat, in terror what that sight might mean,
> I reeled and shivered earthward like a feather

Today I ask for inner strength when difficulties arise.

June 4th

On this day in 1798 the Venetian adventurer and philanderer Giacomo Casanova died. People who are so well known that their own name becomes a term to describe a certain behaviour, are usually successful and respected, even if not liked; Machiavelli for example, or Houdini, or Napoleon.

In the case of Casanova it seems to have been the quantity of his conquests that was remarkable. Apart from the bedroom, he seems to have excelled at very little and to have spent much of his life travelling round a number of European countries, including England, trying to sell them the idea of a National Lottery which, at the time, none of them wanted.

Casanova died aged 73 in Prague, still hoping to ingratiate himself into high society. His last words were: "I have lived as a philosopher and I die as a Christian". Both statements are probably open to question.

This poem by George Crabbe is called *Late Wisdom*:

> We've trod the maze of error round,
>   Long wandering in the winding glade;
> And now the torch of truth is found,
>   It only shows us where we strayed:
> By long experience taught, we know –
>   Can rightly judge of friends and foes;
> Can all the worth of these allow,
>   And all the faults discern in those.
> Now, 'tis our boast that we can quell
>   The wildest passions in their rage,
> Can their destructive force repel,
>   And their impetuous wrath assuage.-
> Ah, Virtue! Dost thou arm when now?
>   This bold rebellious race are fled?
> When all these tyrants rest, and thou
>   Art warring with the mighty dead?

Today I will try to be completely honest with myself.

June 5th

On this day in 1898 the Spanish poet Federico Garcia Lorca was born near Granada, Andalusia. As a student he became friends with Salvador Dali and Luis Bunuel but after his homosexual advances were rejected, they drifted apart. He afterwards took the film that Dali and Bunuel made together – *Un Chien Andalou* (*An Andalusian Dog*), as an attack on himself.

Lorca wrote several successful plays but is remembered chiefly for his avant garde poetry. He was murdered in August 1936 but his body was never found – he was 38 years old.

Here is his poem, Arbolé Arbolé:

Tree, tree,
dry and green.
The girl with the pretty face
is out picking olives.
The wind, playboy of towers,
grabs her around the waist.
Four riders passed by
on Andalusian ponies,
with blue and green jackets
and big, dark capes.
'Come to Cordoba, muchacha.'
The girl won't listen to them.
Three young bullfighters passed,
slender in the waist,
with jackets the color of oranges
and swords of ancient silver.
'Come to Sevilla, muchacha.'

The girl won't listen to them.
When the afternoon had turned
dark brown, with scattered light,
a young man passed by, wearing
roses and myrtle of the moon.
'Come to Granada, muchacha.'
And the girl won't listen to him.
The girl with the pretty face
keeps on picking olives
with the grey arm of the wind
wrapped around her waist.
Tree, tree
dry and green

Today I will try to add a spiritual dimension to my life so that I will never be alone when dealing with life's problems.

June 6th

On this day in 1799 the Russian poet Alexander Pushkin was born. Pushkin was a member of the Russian nobility. By all accounts he was sensitive and quick to take offence; a veteran of 28 duels, the 29th killed him at the age of 38. Many of his verse stories such as Boris Godunov and Eugene Onegin were turned into operas and ballets and his short poetic drama Mozart and Salieri was the inspiration for Peter Shaffer's film Amadeus.

This poem, *A Magic Moment I Remember*, by Pushkin may have been written to any of several ladies – he was a popular man:

> *A magic moment I remember:*
> *I raised my eyes and you were there,*
> *A fleeting vision, the quintessence*
> *Of all that's beautiful and rare*
> *I pray to mute despair and anguish,*
> *To vain the pursuits world esteems,*
> *Long did I hear your soothing accents,*
> *Long did your features haunt my dreams.*
> *Time passed. A rebel storm-blast scattered*
> *The reveries that once were mine*
> *And I forgot your soothing accents,*
> *Your features gracefully divine.*
> *In dark days of enforced retirement*
> *I gazed upon grey skies above*
> *With no ideals to inspire me*
> *No one to cry for, live for, love.*
> *Then came a moment of renaissance,*
> *I looked up – you again are there*
> *A fleeting vision, the quintessence*
> *Of all that's beautiful and rare.*

Today I will remember that today is all the time that I have. I will use it well so that tomorrow will be even better.

June 7th

On this day in 1848 the French painter Paul Gauguin was born in Paris. Gauguin's family moved to Peru a year later and he did not return to France until he was seven. He seems to have been a restless soul who lived in many places with different people. When his mother died he was in the Caribbean with the navy.

He returned to Paris and, for the next 11 years, was a successful stockbroker. However, Gauguin seems to have had a wanderlust that meant he never stayed anywhere for long. His disastrous attempt to share a working relationship with Vincent Van Gogh and his later departure for the South Seas, where he spent his last years, are well known.

At almost the same time, the Scottish writer Robert Louis Stevenson was living on another Pacific island where he wrote this (the two never met as far as we know):

About the sheltered garden ground
The trees stand strangely still.
The vale ne'er seemed so deep before,
Nor yet so high the hill.
An awful sense of quietness,
A fulness of repose
Breathes from the dewy garden-lawns,
The silent garden rows.
As the hoof-beats of a troop of horse
Heard far across a plain,
A nearer knowledge of great thoughts
Thrills vaguely through my brain.
I lean my head upon my arm,
My heart's too full to think;
Like the roar of seas, upon my heart
Doth the morning stillness sink.

Today I will remind myself that success in anything does not come easily – if I want a result, then I have to put in the effort.

June 8th

On this day in 1810 the German composer Robert Schumann was born. During his 46 years he composed a body of musical work that is greatly admired today. His story is however, a sad one.

He was plagued throughout his adult life by mental illness and spent his last two years in a lunatic asylum where he died, it is thought, from a brain tumour. He was happily married to Clara, the daughter of his piano teacher, who was an accomplished concert pianist herself.

Together they befriended the brilliant young composer Johannes Brahms, and since Schumann was also a music critic for leading journals, were able to further his career considerably.

Beautiful music seems to inspire beautiful verses. Here are two examples, the first by Shelley:

Music, when soft voices die,
Vibrates in the memory;
Odours, when sweet violets sicken,
Live within the sense they quicken.
Rose leaves, when the rose is dead,
Are heap'd for the belovèd's bed;
And so thy thoughts, when thou art gone,
Love itself shall slumber on.
And here is part of an equally famous one from Shakespeare:
Orpheus with his lute made trees,
And the mountain tops that freeze,
Bow themselves when he did sing:
To his music plants and flowers
Ever sprung; as sun and showers
There had made a lasting spring.

Today I will be grateful for all the beautiful things in the world, some of which, like music and poetry, are easy to take for granted.

June 9th

On this day in 1870 the English writer Charles Dickens died. The man who wrote the best-selling novel of all time, *A Tale of Two Cities*, was wildly popular in his lifetime, partly because his works were first serialised in popular magazines and journals which made them not only monthly cliff-hangers but also cheap and accessible to the masses.

Famously, when *The Old Curiosity Shop* was being serialised, American fans waited at the New York docks, shouting out to the incoming ship, "Is little Nell dead?" Dickens never forgot his own miserable childhood when he was forced to work in a factory while his father languished in a debtor's prison.

Here is a poem from another work weary Victorian – Christina Georgina Rossetti, *Weary In Well-Doing*:

I would have gone; God bade me stay:

> I would have worked; God bade me rest.
> He broke my will from day to day,
> He read my yearnings unexpressed
> And said them nay.
> Now I would stay; God bids me go:
> Now I would rest; God bids me work.
> He breaks my heart tossed to and fro,
> My soul is wrung with doubts that lurk
> And vex it so.
> I go, Lord, where Thou sendest me;
> Day after day I plod and moil:
> But, Christ my God, when will it be
> That I may let alone my toil
> And rest with Thee?

Today I will do my best in everything that I set out to do because I believe that it is part of my purpose in life, and anything less would be bad for my self-esteem.

June 10th

On this day in BC 323 Alexander the Great, King of Macedonia, Persia and Asia and Pharaoh of Egypt, died aged 32. Historians are divided as to what or who killed him. Certainly he was in poor health already from his many campaigns and had recently indulged in one of his long drinking bouts.

Many historians, including some of the ancients, believe that he was deliberately poisoned while others consider it to be the result of alcoholism. After his death his huge empire fell apart as his lieutenants fought for power and territory.

Here is a poem by James Elroy Flecker about conquest, *War Song of the Saracens*:

Not on silk nor in samet we lie, not in curtained solemnity die
Among women who chatter and cry, and children who mumble a
*   prayer*
"We are they who come faster than fate: we are they who ride early
*   or late:*
We storm at your ivory gate: Pale Kings of the Sunset, beware!
But we sleep by the ropes of the camp, and we rise with a shout, and
*   we tramp*
With the sun or the moon for a lamp, and the spray of the wind in
*   our hair.*
From the lands, where the elephants are, to the forts of Merou and
*   Balghar,*
Our steel we have brought and our star to shine on the ruins of Rum.
We have marched from the Indus to Spain, and by God we will go
*   there again;*
We have stood on the shore of the plain where the Waters of Destiny
*   boom"*

Today I accept that I have no need to be a conqueror of anything except myself.

June 11th

On this day in 1184 BC, according to legend, the ancient city of Troy was sacked. Paris, son of King Priam of Troy, fell in love and captured Helen, wife of Menelaus King of Sparta. Enraged, the Greeks came in force to win her back.

All this is impossible to verify. It seems more likely that the Greek expedition was some kind of trade war because the supposed site of Troy was on the Bosphorus, the great sea trade route between the East and the West.

The legend of Troy is nevertheless one of the world's greatest stories, immortalised by Homer as the Roman poet Horace put it so well:

> Vixere fortes ante Agamemnona
> Multi sed omnes illacrimabiles
> Urgentur ignotique longa
> Nocte carent quia vate sacro.
> (Many great men lived before Agamemnon
> But they all lie through the long night
> Unmourned and unrecognised,
> Because they lacked a sacred bard).

Many subsequent writers have drawn on Homer's work. Here are Marlowe's famous lines from his play *Dr Faustus*:

> Was this the face that launched a thousand ships
> And burnt the topless towers of Ilium?
> Sweet Helen, make me immortal with a kiss. [Kisses her.]
> Her lips suck forth my soul; see where it flies! –
> Come, Helen, come, give me my soul again.
> Here will I dwell, for Heaven is in these lips,
> And all is dross that is not Helena.

Today I will remember Dr Faustus and not allow instant gratification to deflect me from my long term needs.

June 12th

On this day in 1802 Harriet Martineau the English writer and sociologist was born. Martineau's work was admired by Queen Victoria.

She was never afraid to speak her mind and made herself unpopular on a trip to America when she wrote scathingly of the treatment of women and slaves there. Later she visited Egypt and shocked many by opining that there was little difference between the lifestyle of an ancient Egyptian and an English country squire.

Here is part of a poem by Aphra Behn, another strong woman who was not afraid to speak her mind. Her poem is about impotence, *The Disappointment*:

> Her balmy Lips encountring his,
> Their Bodies as their Souls are joyn'd,
> Where both in Transports were confin'd,
> Extend themselves upon the Moss.
> Cloris half dead and breathless lay,
> Her Eyes appear'd like humid Light,
> Such as divides the Day and Night;
> Or falling Stars, whose Fires decay;
> And now no signs of Life she shows,
> But what in short-breath-sighs returns and goes.
> He saw how at her length she lay,
> He saw her rising Bosom bare,
> Her loose thin Robes, through which appear
> A Shape design'd for Love and Play;
> Abandon'd by her Pride and Shame,
> She do's her softest Sweets dispence,
> Offring her Virgin-Innocence
> A Victim to Loves Sacred Flame;
> Whilst th' or'e ravish'd Shepherd lies,
> Unable to perform the Sacrifice.

Today I will not be afraid to speak my mind.

June 13th

O n this day in 1865 the Irish poet William Butler Yeats was born. In 1923 he received the Nobel Prize for literature. Much of his best work came in his last years, including this epitaph written before his death, aged 75: 'Cast a cold eye on life, on death. Horseman, pass by'.

Yeats grew up as part of the Protestant ascendancy in Ireland and was disturbed by the many political changes going on. The family moved to England where he spent most of his life. His poetry is notable for its atmospheric feel, its passion and joy and its use of rhythm and sound, perhaps surprising in a man who was tone deaf.

Here are some lines from *The Wanderings of Oisin*:

> We rode in sorrow, with strong hounds three,
> Bran, Sceolan, and Lomair,
> On a morning misty and mild and fair.
> The mist-drops hung on the fragrant trees,
> And in the blossoms hung the bees.
> We rode in sadness above Lough Lean,
> For our best were dead on Gavra's green.
> O you, with whom in sloping valleys,
> Or down the dewy forest alleys,
> I chased at morn the flying deer,
> With whom I hurled the hurrying spear,
> And heard the foemen's bucklers rattle,
> And broke the heaving ranks of battle!
> And Bran, Sceolan, and Lomair,
> Where are you with your long rough hair?
> You go not where the red deer feeds,
> Nor tear the foemen from their steeds.

Today I will be grateful that I am exploring my own spirituality and the inspiration that I gain from it.

June 14th

On this day in 1381 King Richard II of England met the leaders of the Peasants' Revolt outside London. It was the bravest and most notable thing that he did during his reign. He was aged only 14 at the time.

Through a combination of force and duplicity the revolt was quelled and its leaders executed. Richard's reign never really got any better and he failed to fight off the challenge of Henry Bolingbroke, son of John of Gaunt.

Bolingbroke successfully deposed Richard in 1399 and imprisoned him in Pontefract Castle, where he died the following year, aged 33, apparently from starvation. It was a sad end for a still young king whose reign had begun so well.

Here is the beginning of Byron's famous poem, *The Prisoner of Chillon*; perhaps Richard felt like this during his imprisonment:

> *My hair is grey, but not with years*
> *Nor grew it white in a single night,*
> *As men's have grown from sudden fears:*
> *My limbs are bow'd, though not with toil,*
> *But rusted with a vile repose,*
> *For they have been a dungeon's spoil,*
> *And mine has been the fate of those*
> *To whom the goodly earth and air*
> *Are bann'd, and barr'd – forbidden fare;*
> *But this was for my father's faith*
> *I suffer'd chains and courted death;*
> *That father perish'd at the stake*
> *For tenets he would not forsake;*
> *And for the same his lineal race*
> *In darkness found a dwelling place;*
> *We were seven – who now are one*

Today I will remember that I have the ability to do anything that I set my mind to – the only thing to stop it will be myself.

June 15th

On this day in 1094 Rodrigo Díaz de Vivar, known as El Cid, occupied the town of Valencia. When much of Spain was under Moorish influence, El Cid (The Nobleman, in Spanish) won many battles to drive them out.

He used psychological warfare and unexpected tactics that were sometimes planned in brainstorming sessions with his commanders before battle – a revolutionary ploy at the time. Legend has it that after his death, at the siege of Valencia, his body in full armour was strapped to his horse to lead a charge against the enemy.

Here is a poem by a great Spaniard, Federico Garcia Lorca, *Gacela of the Dark Death*:

> I want to sleep the dream of the apples,
> To withdraw from the tumult of cemeteries.
> I want to sleep the dream of that child
> Who wanted to cut his heart on the high seas.
> I don't want to hear again that the dead do not lose their blood,
> That the putrid mouth goes on asking for water.
> I don't want to learn of the tortures of the grass,
> Nor of the moon with a serpent's mouth
> That labours before dawn.
> I want to sleep awhile,
> Awhile, a minute, a century;
> Cover me at dawn with a veil,
> Because dawn will throw fistfuls of ants at me,
> And wet with hard water my shoes
> So that the pincers of the scorpion slide.
> For I want to sleep the dream of the apples,
> To learn a lament that will cleanse me to earth;
> For I want to live with that dark child
> Who wanted to cut his heart on the high seas.

Today I will do my best in everything and I will not worry about the future.

June 16th

On this day in 1904 all the events in James Joyce's book *Ulysses* took place; it is known as 'Bloomsday' because the book's hero is Leopold Bloom. The day is now celebrated by Joyce's admirers the world over. In Dublin, fans in Edwardian dress retrace the route taken by Bloom as described in the book.

Joyce was a huge admirer of the original epic by Homer and the book roughly follows the various episodes of the original such as Circe, the Sirens, the Lotus Eaters and Cyclops as well as the Hero's return home to Ithaca. Much of the book is in the style of 'stream of consciousness', which Joyce was in the habit of dictating to his then amanuensis (helper) Samuel Beckett.

Once, while dictating in his apartment, a visitor knocked on the door and Joyce shouted 'come in', words that Beckett faithfully recorded and included in the day's script. Joyce later decided to leave them in.

Here is a poem that was written by Joyce. Some critics have unkindly wondered if the plumbing in his apartment was faulty:

> All day I hear the noise of waters
> Making moan,
> Sad as the sea-bird is when, going
> Forth alone,
> He hears the winds cry to the water's
> Monotone.
> The grey winds, the cold winds are blowing
> Where I go.
> I hear the noise of many waters
> Far below.
> All day, all night, I hear them flowing
> To and fro.

Today I will consider the description of prayer as: the lifting up of the heart and mind to God.

June 17th

On this day in 1871 the American lawyer, civil rights activist and poet James Weldon Johnson was born. Johnson was also a diplomat who served as US consul in Venezuela and Nicaragua in the early part of the 20th century.

His poetry was well received and he played a leading part in the so called 'Harlem Renaissance'. His poem *Lift Ev'ry Voice and Sing* was hugely popular among African American people and became an anthem of the NAACP (National Association for the Advancement of Coloured People) for which Johnson worked for many years. He died in 1938 when his car was hit by a train at a level crossing.

Here is one of his sensitive and haunting poems *The Glory of the Day Was in Her Face*, that seems to stay in the memory after reading:

> The glory of the day was in her face,
> The beauty of the night was in her eyes.
> And over all her loveliness, the grace
> Of Morning blushing in the early skies.
> And in her voice, the calling of the dove;
> Like music of a sweet, melodious part.
> And in her smile, the breaking light of love;
> And all the gentle virtues in her heart.
> And now the glorious day, the beauteous night,
> The birds that signal to their mates at dawn,
> To my dull ears, to my tear-blinded sight
> Are one with all the dead, since she is gone.

Today I will remember that I can change my life – not by escaping to a new one that has the old me in it but by changing the old me into a new me.

June 18th

On this day in 1815 the Battle of Waterloo was fought. As the Duke of Wellington later remarked, it was: 'A damned close run thing.' He would certainly know, having fought in at least 24 previous battles in various parts of the world.

It was a tradition of Wellington to name his battles after the place where he had spent the previous night, hence Waterloo. Two nights earlier, the Duchess of Richmond gave a ball and invited many officers, including Wellington. During the evening, he received word that the French were advancing. Not wanting a panic, he sent the officers one by one to their regiments, and finally left himself. Here is the start of Byron's poem *The Eve of Waterloo*:

> There was a sound of revelry by night,
> And Belgium's capital had gathered then
> Her beauty and her chivalry, and bright
> The lamps shone o'er fair women and brave men.
> A thousand hearts beat happily; and when
> Music arose with its voluptuous swell,
> Soft eyes looked love to eyes which spake again,
> And all went merry as a marriage bell;
> But hush! Hark! A deep sound strikes like a rising knell!
> Did ye not hear it? – No; 'twas but the wind,
> Or the car rattling o'er the stony street;
> On with the dance! Let joy be unconfined;
> No sleep till morn, when youth and pleasure meet
> To chase the glowing hours with flying feet.
> But hark! – That heavy sound breaks in once more,
> As if the clouds its echo would repeat;
> And nearer, clearer, deadlier than before;
> Arm! Arm! It is – it is – the cannon's opening roar!

Today, if life is 'a damn close run thing', I recall the serenity prayer.

June 19th

On this day in 1623 the French philosopher, mathematician and writer Blaise Pascal was born. One of the most profound thinkers since the Graeco Roman period, Pascal's great work, the Pensées, or 'thoughts', are a series of meditations on some of the eternal great questions.

However, it was as a mathematician that he became best known in his lifetime; he confounded Descartes with his precocious paper on conical mathematics. Pascal's father was for a time the chief tax collector at Rouen and Pascal designed a number of machines that would add and subtract, in order to help him in his task.

Pascal is thus credited as an inventor of the calculating machine and therefore indirectly, of the computer. He wrote the Pensées in the last years of his life and they were unfinished at his death. They remain one of the greatest expositions of Christianity ever written.

Today's poem is by Gerard Manley Hopkins, *God's Grandeur*:

The world is charged with the grandeur of God.
It will flame out, like shining from shook foil;
It gathers to a greatness, like the ooze of oil
Crushed. Why do men then now not reck his rod?
Generations have trod, have trod, have trod;
And all is seared with trade; bleared, smeared with toil;
And wears man's smudge and shares man's smell: the soil
Is bare now, nor can foot feel, being shod.
And for all this, nature is never spent;
There lives the dearest freshness deep down things;
And though the last lights off the black West went
Oh, morning, at the brown brink eastward, springs –
Because the Holy Ghost over the bent
World broods with warm breast and with ah! Bright wings.

Today I give thanks for the spiritual dimension in my life.

June 20th

On this day in 1887 the German British artist and writer Kurt Schwitters was born. He came to England before World War II and was interned as a German citizen but managed to keep working on his art.

He saw his work as making something new out of what was available and is chiefly known for his collages made out of old printed material and other detritus. Schwitters lived his last years in the Lake District and died poor and generally unknown though his influence has since been acknowledged by major artists, including Robert Rauschenberg and Damien Hirst.

He was never able to return to Germany and died in 1948, one day after being granted British citizenship. Schwitters could be said to be a man who 'hid his light under a bushel'.

A bit like this lovely poem by Katherine Mansfield, *Secret Flowers*:

> Is love a light for me? A steady light,
> A lamp within whose pallid pool I dream
> Over old love-books? Or is it a gleam,
> A lantern coming towards me from afar
> Down a dark mountain? Is my love a star?
> Ah me! – So high above so coldly bright!
> The fire dances. Is my love a fire
> Leaping down the twilight muddy and bold?
> The flower petals fold. They are by the sun
> Forgotten. In a shadowy wood they grow
> Where the dark trees keep up a to-and-fro
> Shadowy waving. Who will watch them shine
> When I have dreamed my dream? Ah, darling mine,
> Find them, gather them for me one by one.

Today I will work to make the best use out of whatever is available both in myself and elsewhere.

June 21st

On this day in 1980 Jean Paul Sartre, philosopher and writer, was born.

A prisoner of war during World War II, he was later active in the French Resistance. He remained a simple man with few possessions, actively committed to causes until the end of his life, such as the strikes in Paris in the summer of 1968 during which he was arrested for civil disobedience. President de Gaulle intervened and pardoned him, commenting that "you don't arrest Voltaire."

Sartre is also remembered for his open relationship with feminist writer Simone de Beauvoir who shared his views but not his apartment – the two would meet for lunch almost every day. They remained a couple for over 50 years. De Beauvoir edited all of Sartre's work, most of which he dedicated to her. His best known quote was: "L'enfer, c'est les autres", usually translated as "Hell is other people" – presumably this did not include de Beauvoir.

Here is a poem by Rabindranath Tagore, *Where the Mind is Without Fear*:

> *Where the mind is without fear and the head is held high*
> *Where knowledge is free*
> *Where the world has not been broken up into fragments*
> *By narrow domestic walls*
> *Where words come out from the depth of truth*
> *Where tireless striving stretches its arms towards perfection*
> *Where the clear stream of reason has not lost its way*
> *Into the dreary desert sand of dead habit*
> *Where the mind is led forward by thee*
> *Into ever-widening thought and action*
> *Into that heaven of freedom, my Father, let my country*
> *awake.*

Today I will remember that I cannot know what is best for others; I can only offer comfort, empathy and example.

June 22nd

On this day in 1898 the German writer Erich Maria Remarque was born. Conscripted into the German army aged 18, he wrote one of the most memorable and certainly one of the bestselling stories of the First World War – *All Quiet On The Western Front*.

Written from the point of view of a German soldier, it is notably without hatred or rancour. Remarque wrote many other books as well, without a similar success. He moved to Switzerland after the war and later became an object of hate to the Nazis, who made wild accusations that he was really a Jew and his name was 'Kramer' spelt backwards. They also said, quite wrongly, that he had never fought in the First World War. This forced him to move to the United States, where he was a popular figure, marrying the film star Paulette Goddard.

Here is a poem by William Blake about doing away with hatred, *A Poison Tree*:

> I was angry with my friend:
> I told my wrath, my wrath did end.
> I was angry with my foe:
> I told it not, my wrath did grow.
> And I watered it in fears,
> Night and morning with my tears;
> And I sunned it with smiles,
> And with soft deceitful wiles.
> And it grew both day and night,
> Till it bore an apple bright.
> And my foe beheld it shine.
> And he knew that it was mine,
> And into my garden stole
> When the night had veiled the pole;
> In the morning glad I see
> My foe outstretched beneath the tree.

Today I will not allow anger to spoil my serenity.

June 23rd

On this day in 1910 the French dramatist Jean Anouilh was born. Much of Anouilh's drama was produced during some of France's darkest days during World War II.

He is perhaps best known for his adaptation of Sophocles' great play Antigone which many saw as an allegory of the moral struggle for the soul of France during the Vichy period.

His famous historical plays are on the theme of moral integrity in a time of compromise and collapse. Although Anouilh foreshadowed later writers such as Beckett and Ionesco, his realism and traditionalist structure eventually put him out of fashion. Here is part of Antigone's great speech on morality, from Sophocles' play:

> *Antigone, speaking to Creon, King of Thebes:*
> *"Yes; for it was not Zeus that published that edict;*
> *The justice of the Gods below and their laws are not thus given to men,*
> *I do not consider that your decrees have such force, that a mere man can override the unwritten and infallible laws of heaven.*
> *For such laws are not of to-day or yesterday, but of all time, and no man knows when they were first issued.*
> *I would be ashamed to answer to the Gods for breaking their laws.*
> *Die I must, – I know that well (how should I not?) – even without your edicts.*
> *But if I am to die before my time, I count that a gain: for when any one lives, as I do, beset about with evils, can one find anything but gain in death? So for me to meet this doom is trifling grief;*
> *But if I had allowed my brother, my mother's son to lie in death an unburied corpse, that would have grieved me more; for my own death I am not grieved.*
> *And if my present deeds are foolish in your sight, it may be that a foolish judge will charge me for such folly."*

Today I give thanks for the brave and fearless people in the world.

June 24th

On this day in 1842 the American critic and writer Ambrose Bierce was born. During his life he was famous for his direct, penetrating style and his spare but vivid descriptions, particularly of war. We know that he was one of 13 children, born in a log cabin in Ohio to well-educated parents who, for reasons unknown, gave all their offspring names that began with the letter 'A'.

This is a lot more than we know about his death at the age of 71; apparently he had travelled to Mexico while researching a book on the Mexican Civil War that was then raging. He was last heard of in the town of Chihuahua and then he just disappeared. Some speculated that his sense of humour had led to him planning his demise.

Here is his quirky poem, *Christian*:

> *I dreamed I stood upon a hill, and, lo!*
> *The godly multitudes walked to and fro*
> *Beneath, in Sabbath garments fitly clad,*
> *With pious mien, appropriately sad,*
> *While all the church bells made a solemn din –*
> *A fire-alarm to those who lived in sin.*
> *Then saw I gazing thoughtfully below,*
> *With tranquil face, upon that holy show*
> *A tall, spare figure in a robe of white,*
> *Whose eyes diffused a melancholy light.*
> *'God keep you, stranger,' I exclaimed. 'You are*
> *No doubt (your habit shows it) from afar;*
> *And yet I entertain the hope that you,*
> *Like these good people, are a Christian too.'*
> *He raised his eyes and with a look so stern*
> *It made me with a thousand blushes burn*
> *Replied – his manner with disdain was spiced:*
> *'What! I a Christian? No, indeed! I'm Christ.'*

Today I will try to be direct and honest in all my dealings.

June 25th

O n this day in 1903 the English writer Eric Blair, whose pen name was George Orwell, was born. His writings gave us some of the best known terms for a dystopian society, such as Big Brother and Room 101, and he wrote some chilling predictions of the future.

Orwell came from a relatively poor family but won a scholarship to Eton. After the Second World War he became known to the wider public through his books of political satire – *Animal Farm* and *Nineteen Eighty-Four*. Most of his life and his writing was given to highlighting the struggles of underprivileged people, as described in his book *Down and out in Paris and London*.

He probably knew this poem by Thomas Hardy about a meeting of struggling people, *At the Railway Station, Upway*:

> There is not much that I can do,
> For I've no money that's quite my own!"
> Spoke up the pitying child –
> A little boy with a violin
> At the station before the train came in, –
> "But I can play my fiddle to you,
> And a nice one 'tis, and good in tone!"
> The man in the handcuffs smiled;
> The constable looked, and he smiled too,
> As the fiddle began to twang;
> And the man in the handcuffs suddenly sang
> With grimful glee: "This life so free is the thing for me!"
> And the constable smiled, and said no word,
> As if unconscious of what he heard;
> And so they went on till the train came in –
> The convict, and boy with the violin.

Today I will remember that there are probably many struggling people around me whom I should try to help.

June 26th

On this day in 1885 the French writer and politician André Maurois was born. Maurois spent time in Britain before the fall of France in 1940 and was a pronounced Anglophile who wrote biographies of Disraeli, Dickens, Shelley and Byron as well as Balzac, George Sand and Victor Hugo.

A French Academician, he moved to America to work against Nazi propaganda. Born Émile Herzog, he changed his name to André Maurois in 1947.

Here is a poem by the English poet that Maurois most admired – Percy Bysshe Shelley, *Love's Philosophy*:

> The fountains mingle with the river,
> And the rivers with the ocean;
> The winds of heaven mix forever
> With a sweet emotion;
> Nothing in the world is single;
> All things by a law divine
> In another's being mingle –
> Why not I with thine?
> See, the mountains kiss high heaven,
> And the waves clasp one another;
> No sister flower could be forgiven
> If it disdained its brother;
> And the sunlight clasps the earth,
> And the moonbeams kiss the sea –
> What are all these kissings worth,
> If thou kiss not me?

Today I will remember the words of André Maurois: Often we allow ourselves to be upset by small things we should despise and forget.

June 27th

On this day in 1887 Helen Keller met Annie Sullivan. Helen Keller was rendered deaf and blind by an illness (possibly meningitis) at the age of 19 months. Sullivan finally achieved a breakthrough, when Keller felt running water and recognised the connection with the symbol pressed into her other hand.

By 1900 Keller had gained admittance to Radcliffe College. She wrote several books and campaigned for the rights of disadvantaged people. She died in 1968 aged 87. Helen Keller said of poetry: "Great poetry, whether written in Greek or in English, needs no other interpreter than a responsive heart." When Annie died in 1936, Helen Keller was holding her hand. There are many statues of Keller and Sullivan. One bears the inscription: "The best and most beautiful things in the world cannot be seen or even touched, they must be felt with the heart."

Elizabeth Barrett Browning's sonnet says something similar, in her Sonnets from the Portuguese:

> When our two souls stand up erect and strong,
> Face to face, silent, drawing nigh and nigher,
> Until the lengthening wings break into fire
> At either curvèd point, – what bitter wrong
> Can the earth do to us, that we should not long
> Be here contented? Think. In mounting higher,
> The angels would press on us, and aspire
> To drop some golden orb of perfect song
> Into our deep, dear silence. Let us stay
> Rather on earth, Belovèd, – where the unfit
> Contrarious moods of men recoil away
> And isolate pure spirits, and permit
> A place to stand and love in for a day,
> With darkness and the death-hour rounding it.

Today I will remember that true love consists of giving to others.

June 28th

On this day in 1491 the future King Henry VIII of England was born. His attempts to divorce his first wife, Catherine of Aragon, led to the English Reformation. Catherine steadfastly refused a divorce and probably continued to hold him in high regard despite his behaviour.

Perhaps because of the early death of his older brother , he was obsessed with the succession, in what came to be known at court as 'The King's Great Matter'. This led him to take in all, six wives, two of whom were beheaded for adultery. This lovely anonymous poem was probably written not long after Henry's death. It could have been penned by Catherine of Aragon, *Since First I saw your Face*:

> *Since first I saw your face I resolv'd*
> *To honour and renown you;*
> *If now I be disdain'd I wish*
> *My heart had never known you.*
> *What I that loved and you that liked,*
> *Shall we begin to wrangle?*
> *No, no, no! my heart is fast*
> *And cannot disentangle.*
> *The Sun, whose beams most glorious are,*
> *Rejecteth no beholder,*
> *And your sweet beauty past compare,*
> *Made my poor eyes the bolder:*
> *Where beauty moves and wit delights,*
> *And signs of kindness bind me,*
> *There, oh there! Where e'er I go*
> *I leave my heart behind me.*
> *If I desire or praise you too much,*
> *That fault you may forgive me;*
> *Or if my hands had strayed but a touch,*
> *Then justly might you leave me*

Today I will be true and steadfast in all my relationships.

June 29th

On this day in 1861 the English writer and poet Elizabeth Barrett Browning died, aged 55. Considered one of the leading poets of the Victorian era, she suffered from ill health for most of her life and after marrying Robert Browning in 1846, lived in Italy where she grew stronger and bore a son.

Elizabeth's family owned plantations in Jamaica, and though this was the source of much wealth, she became an abolitionist campaigner and a promoter of women's rights. Her poetry was so well regarded that she was in contention to become Poet Laureate at one time (the post was given to Tennyson).

Here is an example from her work *Sonnets From The Portuguese* (Browning used to call her 'My little Portuguese'),

How Do I Love Thee?

How do I love thee? Let me count the ways.
I love thee to the depth and breadth and height
My soul can reach, when feeling out of sight
For the ends of being and ideal grace.
I love thee to the level of every day's
Most quiet need, by sun and candle-light.
I love thee freely, as men strive for right.
I love thee purely, as they turn from praise.
I love thee with the passion put to use
In my old griefs, and with my childhood's faith.

Today I will not wear a mask and I will show my true emotions.

June 30th

On this day in 1685 the English poet and dramatist John Gay was born. Gay seems to have been a man who made friends easily and was able to find patrons for his work in spite of their somewhat risqué nature.

He is best known for his play *The Beggar's Opera* which is a thinly veiled satire criticising the government of the day under Robert Walpole. Gay is buried at Westminster Abbey. The epitaph that he wrote for himself is suitably wry: 'Life is a jest, and all things show it, I thought so once, and now I know it.'

Here is one of his poems – *Elegy on a Lap Dog*:

> Shock's fate I mourn; poor Shock is now no more,
>   Ye Muses mourn, ye chamber-maids deplore.
> Unhappy Shock! Yet more unhappy fair,
>   Doom'd to survive thy joy and only care!
>   Thy wretched fingers now no more shall deck,
> And tie the fav'rite ribbon round his neck;
> No more thy hand shall smooth his glossy hair,
> And comb the wavings of his pendent ear.
>   Yet cease thy flowing grief, forsaken maid;
> All mortal pleasures in a moment fade:
>   Our surest hope is in an hour,
> And love, best gift of heav'n, not long enjoy'd.
>   Methinks I see her frantic with despair,
>   Her streaming eyes, wrung hands, and flowing hair
> Her Mechlen pinners rent the floor bestrow,
>   And her torn fan gives real signs of woe.
>   Hence Superstition, that tormenting guest,
>   That haunts with fancied fears the coward breast;
>   No dread events upon his fate attend,
>   Stream eyes no more, no more thy tresses rend

Today I will be grateful that I have feelings that I can recognise.

July 1st

On this day in 1804 the French writer Amantine Lucile Aurore Dudevant (née Dupin), whose pseudonym was George Sand, was born. This rebellious, cross-dressing, cigar-smoking woman is remembered today less for her writing than for being herself; the freedom that she represented, the boundaries that she completely ignored, the propriety she didn't care about, the lives she changed.

Romantically linked to many famous names in the world of art and culture, including Chopin, Liszt and de Musset, she fearlessly cut a swathe through male chauvinist attitudes, at least a century ahead of her time. She is a shining embodiment of the maxim 'know thyself – be thyself' and women today have much to thank her for. The world today likes conformity. Idiosyncratic people may be tolerated and even admired at times, but we can't handle too many of them. Yet we are all unique and should strive to be ourselves.

Today's poem is part of a longer work, *The Holy Office* by James Joyce; I think it describes George Sand rather well:

> *So distantly I turn to view*
> *The shamblings of that motley crew,*
> *Those souls that hate the strength that mine has*
> *Steeled in the school of old Aquinas.*
> *Let them continue as is meet*
> *To adequate the balance-sheet.*
> *Though they may labour to the grave*
> *My spirit shall they never have*
> *Nor make my soul with theirs as one*
> *Till the Mahamanvantara be done:*
> *And though they spurn me from their door*
> *My soul shall spurn them evermore.*

Today I will strive to know myself and be true to myself, whatever others may say.

July 2nd

On this day in 1961 the author Ernest Hemingway died by his own hand – he used his favourite shotgun. One of the greatest writers of the 20th century, Hemingway wrote many memorable books. Two of them in particular, *For Whom the Bell Tolls* and *A Farewell to Arms*, are about strong men in harsh and dangerous situations.

He was a lover of bullfighting, hunting, big game fishing and skiing. Much of his life involved struggling with his own demons – and it showed in the form of heavy drinking and bouts of depression.

Very few people show their true selves consistently in what they do and what they say. A lot of us want to hide the truth in case it might show us in a bad light. The problem with doing this is that others don't get to see who we really are and thus can't give us the help that we may need. In his troubled family, Hemingway's father and two of his siblings also committed suicide. Although Hemingway can be said to have lived life to the full, it seems that he couldn't live with himself.

This poem, *The Touch* by James Graham, Marquis of Montrose (executed in 1650 for treason) is about living life to the full:

> He either fears his fate too much,
> Or his deserts are small,
> That puts it not unto the touch,
> To win or lose it all.

And here is fellow Scot Robert Burns' *Epigram on a Suicide*:

> Earthed up, here lies an imp o' hell,
> Planted by Satan's dibble;
> Poor silly wretch, he's damned himsel',
> To save the lord the trouble.

Today I will remember those in emotional distress.

July 3rd

On this day in 1886, the first motor car was driven in Germany by Karl Benz. With more than a billion cars in the world now, it is hard to imagine what it was like in 1886.

Life followed a simpler pattern. This meant that people had more time – for helping and understanding each other. On the other hand, travel was much more tiring and emergency services – police, ambulance and fire brigade – were less reliable.

Driving a motor car is putting oneself inside a steel carapace and cutting oneself off from other people. However useful a motor car may be, it does not contribute much to general understanding and communication between people.

Today's poem, by Henry Lawson, has a flavour of that. Though written roughly one hundred years ago, it could apply to people today:

The Lady of the motor car, she stareth straight ahead;
Her face is like the stone, my friend, her face is like the dead;
Her face is like the living dead, because she is "well-bred" –
Because her heart is dead, my friend, as all her life was dead.
The Lady in her motor car, she speaketh like a man,
Because her girlhood never was, nor womanhood began.
She says, "To the Aus-traliah, John!" and "Home" when she hath been.
And to the husband at her side she says, "Whhat doo you mean?"
The Lady of the motor car, her very soul is dead,
Because she never helped herself nor had to work for bread;
The Lady of the motor car sits in her sitting-room,
Her stony face has never changed though all the land is gloom.

Today I will not cut myself off from other people – I will try to communicate and to understand others.

July 4th

On this day in 1776 the US congress proclaimed the Declaration of Independence from Britain. There is not much more about this event that hasn't already been said. Post-Columbian America only has five hundred odd years of history. However, it doesn't seem to worry Americans.

Whatever sense of national identity they lack compared to, say, Egypt (at least five thousand years of history), they make up for in energy and imagination. It must have taken courage on that day to defy one of the then greatest countries in the world by signing the Declaration. As Benjamin Franklin said to his 55 co-signatories: "we must all hang together or assuredly we will all hang separately."

Today's poem is by Englishman George Crabbe who lived at the time of the War of Independence, *Late Wisdom*:

> We've trod the maze of error round,
>   Long wandering in the winding glade;
> And now the torch of truth is found,
>   It only shows us where we strayed:
> By long experience taught, we know –
>   Can rightly judge of friends and foes;
> Can all the worth of these allow,
>   And all the faults discern in those.
> Now, 'tis our boast that we can quell
>   The wildest passions in their rage,
> Can their destructive force repel,
>   And their impetuous wrath assuage.-
> Ah, Virtue! Dost thou arm when now
>   This bold rebellious race are fled?
> When all these tyrants rest, and thou
>   Art warring with the mighty dead?

Today I ask for the courage to change the things I can.

July 5th

On this day in 1861 the first speed limit was introduced in Great Britain – of 10 mph (16 km/h) on open roads, reduced to 2 mph (3 km/h) in towns.

The first person to be convicted of speeding is believed to be Walter Arnold of East Peckham, Kent who, in 1896, was fined for speeding at 8 mph (13 km/h).

This ditty from the early 20th century typifies the drivers of the time:

> *I collided with some trippers*
> *In my swift de Dion Bouton*
> *Squashed them out as flat as kippers*
> *Left them "aussi mort que mouton".*
> *What a nuisance trippers are*
> *I must now repaint my car.*

Motoring was a different experience before the advent of the motorway in the 1940s. Driving seemed to be altogether more light-hearted.

Here is an extract from a 1931 book, *Adele & Co* by Dornford Yates, a writer whose thrillers in their day were almost as popular as John Buchan's:

> "We shot up the hill, whipped through a grove of chestnuts and tore down a long, straight stretch at 85. As I steadied her up for the corner, one mile was gone. We flung around the bend and another, brushed some hay from a wagon and slashed a thicket in two. For a furlong we swam between meadows. Then we switched to the right and leapt at a ridge."
> It was a different era.

Today I pray for all motorists, that their journeys may be safe for them and for others.

July 6th

On this day in 1935 His Holiness the 14th Dalai Lama, Tenzin Gyatso was born. The spiritual leader of Tibet came from a farming family in north-eastern Tibet and was recognised as the reincarnation of the Dalai Lama at the age of two.

Describing himself as a simple Buddhist monk, he has received numerous honours and awards including the 1989 Nobel peace prize. He travels widely and is a passionate advocate of his three main commitments in life: the promotion of basic human values; the promotion of harmony and understanding among the world's major religions; and the welfare of the Tibetan people.

The Dalai Lama is a shining example of simplicity and acceptance of one's lot, as echoed in this poem by 17th century poet Thomas Dekker, *O Sweet Content*:

> *Art thou poor, yet hast thou golden slumbers?*
> *O sweet content!*
> *Art thou rich, yet is thy mind perplex'd?*
> *O punishment!*
> *Dost thou laugh to see how fools are vex'd*
> *To add to golden numbers, golden numbers?*
> *O sweet content! O sweet, O sweet content!*
> *Work apace, apace, apace, apace;*
> *Honest labour bears a lovely face;*
> *Then hey nonny nonny, hey nonny nonny!*
> *Canst drink the waters of the crispèd spring?*
> *O sweet content!*
> *Swimm'st thou in wealth, yet sink'st in thine own tears?*
> *O punishment!*
> *Then he that patiently want's burden bears*
> *No burden bears, but in a king, a king!*
> *O sweet content! O sweet, O sweet content!*

Today I will seek simplicity and acceptance.

July 7th

On this date in 1550 chocolate was introduced to Europe from the Americas. There is evidence that the peoples of Central America used chocolate as a drink as early as 1900 BC. Christopher Columbus reports finding it during his fourth expedition in 1502.

The Maya and Aztec people considered it a delicacy and the emperor Montezuma is described enjoying it by a Spanish observer, Antonio de Solis: "When he had done eating, he usually took a Kind of Chocolate, made after the Manner of the Country, that is, the Substance of the Nut beat up with the Mill till the Cup was filled more with Froth than with Liquor; after which he used to smoak Tobacco perfum'd with liquid Amber."

Production of chocolate was gradually refined throughout the 18th century to make it less bitter to taste; further processes in the 19th century transformed it into solid form. Today hundreds millions of tons of chocolate are consumed each year worldwide, and the average consumption per person in the UK exceeds 11 kilos per year. The negative impact on health from overindulgence is thought to be very considerable.

Poet Andrew Marvell's *The Garden* has this juicy stanza:

> *What wondrous life is this I lead!*
> *Ripe apples drop about my head;*
> *The luscious clusters of the vine*
> *Upon my mouth do crush their wine;*
> *The nectarine and curious peach*
> *Into my hands themselves do reach;*
> *Stumbling on melons as I pass,*
> *Insnared with flowers, I fall on grass.*

Today I ask that I will practise moderation in all things and I will be grateful for the pleasures in life, especially chocolate.

July 8th

On this day in 2011 Betty Ford, First Lady to US President Gerald Ford, died. She was a well-liked and outspoken figure on subjects such as the feminist movement, and civil rights. Perhaps what she will be remembered for most is the establishment of the Betty Ford Centre for Addiction Recovery, following her admission and successful treatment for alcoholism and substance abuse in 1978. Betty Ford did much to alleviate the stigma of addiction by talking openly about her experiences in a sensible, no nonsense manner.

Today's poem is by Parisian Charles Baudelaire, a man familiar to the bottle, *Be Drunk*:

Nothing else matters:
That is the only matter.
If you would not feel
Time's horrible burden
Weighing on your shoulders
And crushing you to the earth,
Be drunk all of the time.
And if sometimes,
You should awaken
And the drunkenness be half or wholly slipped away from you,
Ask of the wind,
Or of the wave,
Or of the star,
Or of the bird,
Or of the clock,
Or of whatever flies, or sighs, or rocks, or sings, or speaks,
Ask what hour it is;
And the wind, wave, star, bird,
Clock will answer you:
"It is the hour to be drunk!"

Today I ask for the honesty and common sense to face up to my problems and take responsibility for dealing with them.

July 9th

On this day in 1955 the recording *Rock around the Clock* by Bill Haley and His Comets reached number one in the US Billboard listings. It was not the first rock and roll record, nevertheless it is widely considered to be the song that brought rock and roll into mainstream culture around the world.

Rock and Roll moved on to Elvis, Little Richard and others. Bill Haley and His Comets were soon left behind, but they started it all. Haley died alone in 1981, in the shed at the end of his garden where he lived relatively unknown. He was well aware that people thought of him as avuncular and a little embarrassing, but Pop owes him a great debt.

Today's poem is the original Shaker tune for which *Lord of the Dance* was later written. Simple Gifts was written by Elder Joseph while he was at the Shaker community in Alfred, Maine. The Shakers were an 18th century religious sect who encouraged dancing as a form of prayer. These are the lyrics (I wonder if Bill Haley ever heard them):

> 'Tis the gift to be simple, 'tis the gift to be free
> 'Tis the gift to come down where we ought to be,
> And when we find ourselves in the place just right,
> 'Twill be in the valley of love and delight.
> When true simplicity is gained,
> To bow and to bend we shan't be ashamed,
> To turn, turn will be our delight,
> Till by turning, turning we come 'round right.

Today I ask to accept change positively and to enjoy the new experiences that it brings.

July 10th

On this day in 1040 Lady Godiva rode naked on horseback through Coventry. According to legend, she wanted to force her husband, the Earl of Mercia, to lower taxes. A great story, but there is very little evidence that this actually happened.

On the other hand, perhaps it did. Certainly the story has lasted a long time and become the inspiration for many works of art, including paintings and sculptures. If it did happen, then clearly the lady was way ahead of her time. This story has inspired today's charity fund raisers who do outrageous things to raise money.

Lord Tennyson was inspired to write this poem, *Lady Godiva* 'while waiting for his train in Coventry':

> *Then she rode forth, clothed on with chastity:*
> *The deep air listen'd round her as she rode,*
> *And all the low wind hardly breathed for fear.*
> *The little wide-mouth'd heads upon the spout*
> *Had cunning eyes to see: the barking cur*
> *Made her cheek flame; her palfrey's foot-fall shot*
> *Light horrors thro' her pulses; the blind walls*
> *Were full of chinks and holes; and overhead*
> *Fantastic gables, crowding, stared: but she*
> *Not less thro' all bore up, till, last, she saw*
> *The white-flower'd elder-thicket from the field,*
> *Gleam thro' the Gothic archway in the wall.*
> *Then she rode back, clothed on with chastity;*
> *. . . she took the tax away*
> *And built herself an everlasting name.*

Today I ask that I will be ready to act for causes in which I believe, no matter what the cost to me.

July 11th

On this day in 1690, The Battle of the Boyne was fought between two rival claimants of the English, Scottish, and Irish thrones – the Catholic James II and the Protestant William III. The battle, won by William, was a turning point in James's unsuccessful attempt to regain the crown. This pivotal moment for the Protestant ascendancy in Ireland has been marked ever since, with marching, rioting and other violence.

The battle is nowadays commemorated on the twelfth of July and remains the most important day in the 'marching season' in Northern Ireland. The Peace Process has seen success over the past decade and the hope is that this will continue.

This poem by Arthur Hugh Clough refers to the struggle for peace, *Say not the Struggle nought Availeth*:

> Say not the struggle nought availeth,
> > The labour and the wounds are vain,
> The enemy faints not, nor faileth,
> > And as things have been they remain.
> If hopes were dupes, fears may be liars;
> > It may be, in yon smoke concealed,
> Your comrades chase e'en now the fliers,
> > And, but for you, possess the field.
> For while the tired waves, vainly breaking
> > Seem here no painful inch to gain,
> Far back through creeks and inlets making,
> > Came, silent, flooding in, the main.
> And not by eastern windows only,
> > When daylight comes, comes in the light,
> In front the sun climbs slow, how slowly,
> > But westward, look, the land is bright.

Today I ask that I will be quick to forgive those who have hurt me.

July 12th

On this day in 100 BC Julius Caesar, a politician and a general, was born. Nearly two thousand years later, the name of this man still stands for power and military success. At that time Rome was a republic and the greatest power in the Mediterranean. The conquests and excesses of the empire were still to come.

In 55 BC he invaded Britain as part of his campaign in Gaul, of which he was governor. However, his main goal was always political supremacy at home and, returning with an army in 49 BC, he won the ensuing civil war and had himself declared Dictator.

In 44 BC he had himself declared Dictator for life, but this proved too much for his enemies. In the same year he was assassinated. Shakespeare tells us in his play Julius Caesar how a man who once bestrode the narrow world like a Colossus was laid low by treachery and how death equalises us all.

Here is part of the great speech by Mark Anthony from the play:

Friends, Romans, countrymen, lend me your ears;
I come to bury Caesar, not to praise him.
The evil that men do lives after them;
The good is oft interred with their bones;
So let it be with Caesar. The noble Brutus
Hath told you Caesar was ambitious:
If it were so, it was a grievous fault,
And grievously hath Caesar answer'd it.
You all did love him once, not without cause:
What cause withholds you then, to mourn for him?
O judgment! Thou art fled to brutish beasts,
And men have lost their reason. Bear with me;
My heart is in the coffin there with Caesar,
And I must pause till it come back to me

Today I ask that I will not allow my ambition to influence the choices that I make each day.

July 13th

On this day in 1792 Louis XVI and Marie Antoinette, King and Queen of France, were deposed and imprisoned in Paris. Marie Antoinette married at 15 and the shy Louis reportedly did not consummate the marriage for seven years, giving rise to the popular comment: 'wedded, unbedded and beheaded'.

Probably neither Louis nor his wife were wicked people, but their blatant hedonism quickly alienated the starving masses. Their trials and executions by guillotine the following year was an inevitable conclusion.

Today's poem is an excerpt from *The Flower Girl and the Queen* by Carrie Bell Sinclair:

> *Who is that pale yet stately one,*
> *Robb'd of her royal pride?*
> *The throne, the crown, all from her gone –*
> *The sceptre thrown aside?*
> *Is this the haughty Austrian*
> *That meets each scornful glance?*
> *And will she never reign again*
> *As the proud Queen of France?*
> *Alas! poor, hapless one! thy brow*
> *Is furrowed o'er with care –*
> *For grief has made thy form to bow,*
> *And silvered o'er thy hair!*
> *Still proud, though not in royal robes,*
> *In truth and virtue strong –*
> *Her only prayer for mercy this,*
> *"Don't make me suffer long!"*

Today I ask that pride will not lead me into a false sense of my own importance.

July 14th

On this day in 1846 Henry David Thoreau was jailed in Massachusetts for non-payment of taxes. This event happened while he was engaged in his famous two year experiment of living alone on a hut in the woods so as to experience life and survival at its most basic level.

A Harvard graduate and a free thinker, Thoreau also originated the idea of civil disobedience, arguing that individuals should not allow governments to overrule their consciences and that indeed they have a duty not to allow themselves to be made the agents of injustice. He was motivated at the time by his disgust with slavery but his idea has stood the test of time and has been used in many causes worldwide. Martin Luther King is a famous example.

Today's quote comes from another brave man: Martin Niemöller (1892–1984), a prominent Protestant pastor who emerged as an outspoken public foe of Adolf Hitler and spent the last seven years of Nazi rule in concentration camps. He narrowly escaped execution and lived to become a leading member of the German Peace Movement after the war. He died in Wiesbaden aged 92:

> First they came for the Socialists, and I did not speak out –
> Because I was not a Socialist.
> Then they came for the Trade Unionists, and I did not speak out –
> Because I was not a Trade Unionist.
> Then they came for the Jews, and I did not speak out –
> Because I was not a Jew.
> Then they came for me – and there was no one left to speak for me.

Today I pray that I will be brave enough to speak out whenever I see injustice.

July 15th

On this day in 1799 the Rosetta Stone was found in a village in Egypt. Essentially a large stone inscribed with a decree issued at Memphis in Egypt in 196 BC on behalf of King Ptolemy V, it was discovered by an officer in the army of Napoleon, who had recently invaded Egypt.

It had been used as building material for a military fort. The decree appears in three scripts: ancient Egyptian hieroglyphs, demotic Greek script and ancient Greek. Because it presents essentially the same text in all three scripts, it provides the key to understanding Egyptian hieroglyphs.

Without this astonishing find, our knowledge of life in ancient Egypt would be much more limited. I find it comforting that ancient Egyptians felt like we do.

Consider this Egyptian love poem, written thousands of years ago, *My Heart Flutters Hastily*:

> *My heart flutters hastily,*
> *When I think of my love of you;*
> *It lets me not act sensibly,*
> *It leaps from its place.*
> *It lets me not put on a dress,*
> *Nor wrap my scarf around me;*
> *I put no paint upon my eyes,*
> *I'm even not anointed.*
> *"Don't wait, go there," says it to me,*
> *As often as I think of him;*
> *My heart, don't act so stupidly,*
> *Why do you play the fool?*
> *Sit still, the brother comes to you,*
> *And many eyes as well.*
> *Let not the people say of me:*
> *"A woman fallen through love!"*
> *Be steady when you think of him,*
> *My heart, do not flutter!*

Today I will remember the family to which I belong.

July 16th

On this day in 1951 the novel *The Catcher in the Rye* was published. Teenagers everywhere related to the angst of its young hero, Holden Caulfield. Though written over 60 years ago, it still has a contemporary feel. The author, JD Salinger, never published another full length novel and gradually withdrew from society, dying as a recluse in 2010.

Here is part of a poem, *Genius* by Mark Twain whose Huck Finn can be seen as a forerunner of Holden Caulfield:

Genius, like gold and precious stones,
Is chiefly prized because of its rarity.
Geniuses are people who dash off weird, wild,
Incomprehensible poems with astonishing facility,
And get booming drunk and sleep in the gutter.
Genius elevates its possessor to ineffable spheres
Far above the vulgar world and fills his soul
With regal contempt for the gross and sordid things of earth.
If you see a young man who has frowsy hair
And distraught look, and affects eccentricity in dress,
You may set him down for a genius.
If he is too proud to accept assistance,
And spurns it with a lordly air
At the very same time
That he knows he can't make a living to save his life,
He is most certainly a genius.
If he hangs on and sticks to poetry,
Notwithstanding sawing wood comes handier to him,
He is a true genius.

Today I ask that I will not isolate myself from others but instead I will learn from them.

July 17th

On this day in 1717 the first performance of Handel's Water Music was given, on the River Thames in London. The first performance is recorded in the newspapers of the time. At about 8 pm, King George I and several aristocrats boarded a royal barge at Whitehall Palace for an excursion up the River Thames.

Another barge followed, containing about 50 musicians. Many Londoners also took to the river to hear the concert so that: "the whole River in a manner was covered with boats and barges". On arriving at Chelsea, the King left his barge for a while, returning at about 11pm.

The king was so pleased with the Water Music that he ordered it to be repeated at least three times, both on the trip upstream to Chelsea and on the return, until he landed again at Whitehall. The piece is said to have restored Handel to royal favour.

Here are the words of two of his great Coronation Anthems, taken from scripture:

> *Zadok the Priest and Nathan the Prophet,*
> *Anointed Solomon king.*
> *And all rejoiced and said:*
> *God save the King, long live the King,*
> *May the king live forever! Amen, Alleluia.*
> *(Kings 1:39-40)*

> *The king shall rejoice in thy strength, O Lord!*
> *Exceeding glad shall he be of thy salvation.*
> *Glory and worship has thou laid upon him.*
> *Thou hast presented him with the blessing of goodness*
> *And has set a crown of pure gold upon his head.*
> *(Psalm 21)*

Today I ask that I may take time to enjoy and be grateful for both music and poetry.

July 18th

On this day in 1290 King Edward I of England expelled all Jews from the country and on the same day in 1925, Adolf Hitler in Germany, published *Mein Kampf*. On a day when Hitler took a significant step towards furthering his policies for the establishment of a master race in Germany, we might pause to reflect that at an earlier time, an English King played a part in the sad and long history of Jewish persecution.

England was also the first country to require all Jews to wear a badge denoting their race. Jews were not allowed back into England until Oliver Cromwell ruled the country, in 1657.

By way of contrast, no expulsions ever took place in Scotland, which is thought to have the distinction of being the only European country with no history of state persecution of Jews.

Today's quotation is from Shylock's great speech in Shakespeare's *Merchant of Venice*:

> Hath not a Jew eyes? Hath not a Jew hands, organs,
> Dimensions, senses, affections, passions; fed with
> The same food, hurt with the same weapons, subject
> To the same diseases, healed by the same means,
> Warm'd and cool'd by the same winter and summer
> As a Christian is? If you prick us, do we not bleed?
> If you tickle us, do we not laugh? If you poison us,
> Do we not die? And if you wrong us, shall we not revenge?
> If we are like you in the rest, we will resemble you in that.
> If a Jew wrong a Christian, what is his humility?
> Revenge. If a Christian wrong a Jew, what should his
> Sufferance be by Christian example? Why, revenge.
> The villainy you teach me, I will execute,
> And it shall go hard but I will better the instruction.

Today I ask that I will treat all men as my brothers regardless of race or creed.

July 19th

On this day in 1545 the *Mary Rose*, flagship of the English navy, sank off the Isle of Wight. The English King, Henry VIII was watching. One wonders what he thought. History does not record what he said.

The *Mary Rose* was fighting off a French invasion fleet when she sank and the reason for this is still not properly understood. It is probable that the ship was incorrectly balanced and top heavy with the weight of cannon and other guns and men.

The Mary Rose debacle was a disaster at the time. 73 men died as the ship rapidly sank. In 1982 the remains of the ship were lifted from the sea and carefully restored at Portsmouth, where they are now on display, giving a fascinating example of naval shipboard life of the time.

Today's poem by American Walt Whitman is about seafaring and its dangers, *Aboard at a Ship's Helm*:

Aboard at a ship's helm,
A young steersman steering with care.
Through fog on a sea-coast dolefully ringing,
An ocean-bell – O a warning bell, rock'd by the waves.
O you give good notice indeed, you bell by the sea-reefs ringing,
Ringing, ringing, to warn the ship from its wreck-place.
For as on the alert O steersman, you mind the loud admonition,
The bows turn, the freighted ship tacking speeds away under her
    gray sails,
The beautiful and noble ship with all her precious wealth speeds
Away gayly and safe.
But O the ship, the immortal ship! O ship aboard the ship!
Ship of the body, ship of the soul, voyaging, voyaging, voyaging

Today I ask that I will be helped to steer the ship of my soul on a steady course.

July 20th

O n this day in 356 BC Alexander the Great, King of Macedonia, was born. Alexander changed the face of the civilised world by conquering an area that stretched from Greece eastwards to what is present day Pakistan, including Egypt.

As a youth Alexander was tutored by Aristotle who taught him philosophy, politics and rhetoric as well as introducing him to Homer. The young king was inspired by the story of Achilles and the fall of Troy and carried a copy of Homer's *Iliad* with him wherever he went.

Famous for his drunken orgies as well as his conquests, Alexander fell ill after a heavy drinking session at Persepolis and died in mysterious circumstances, perhaps related to alcoholism. Like his hero Achilles, he had his fatal weakness. There is something unique about Greek history and the poet Ella Wheeler Wilcox probably felt it when she wrote this poem, *At Eleusis*:

> I, at Eleusis, saw the finest sight,
> When early morning's banners were unfurled.
> From high Olympus, gazing on the world,
> The ancient gods once saw it with delight.
> Sad Demeter had in a single night
> Removed her sombre garments! And mine eyes
> Beheld a 'broidered mantle in pale dyes
> Thrown o'er her throbbing bosom. Sweet and clear
> There fell the sound of music on mine ear.
> And from the South came Hermes, he whose lyre
> One time appeased the great Apollo's ire.
> The rescued maid, Persephone, by the hand
> He led to waiting Demeter, and cheer
> And light and beauty once more blessed the land.

Today I seek to be aware of my weaknesses and not allow them to spoil my life, as Alexander may have done.

July 21st

On this day in 1796 Scottish poet Robert Burns died at the age of 37. Burns is widely regarded as the national poet of Scotland and is celebrated worldwide. A pioneer of the Romantic movement, after his death he became a great source of inspiration to the founders of both liberalism and socialism, and a cultural icon in Scotland and among the Scottish Diaspora around the world.

Born in a humble cottage in Ayrshire, he worked in the Customs Service, travelling throughout Scotland and proving once again that great poets can often have mundane day jobs (Philip Larkin was a librarian, TS Eliot worked in a bank).

Today's quote comes from one of his favourite songs, that was originally a bawdy folk song but which Burns rewrote as a tender expression of simple love and friendship:

> *John Anderson my jo, John,*
> *   When we were first acquent;*
> *Your locks were like the raven,*
> *   Your bony brow was brent;*
> *But now your brow is beld, John,*
> *   Your locks are like the snaw;*
> *But blessings on your frosty pow,*
> *   John Anderson my Jo.*
> *John Anderson my jo, John,*
> *   We clamb the hill the gither;*
> *And mony a canty day, John,*
> *   We've had wi' ane anither:*
> *Now we maun totter down, John,*
> *   And hand in hand we'll go;*
> *And sleep the gither at the foot,*
> *   John Anderson my Jo.*

Today I ask that I will be grateful for the friendships that have enriched my life.

July 22nd

On this day in 1893 the famous song *America the Beautiful* was written by Katharine Lee Bates, following a trip to the Rocky Mountains. Bates was an academic who spent most of her life teaching in Massachusetts, where she died aged 69.

America the Beautiful, with its stirring tune, has become an unofficial national anthem which anyone who has visited that country can respond to. It stresses the beauty and freedom of that great country but it makes no mention of the millions of African slaves and Native Americans who suffered. Anthems are like that and it would be unreasonable to expect otherwise. It does not mean that we should never look inside the façade.

Here is a fragment:

> O beautiful for spacious skies,
> For amber waves of grain,
> For purple mountain majesties
> Above the fruited plain!
> America! America!
> God shed his grace on thee
> And crown thy good with brotherhood
> From sea to shining sea!
>
> O beautiful for pilgrim feet
> Whose stern impassioned stress
> A thoroughfare of freedom beat
> Across the wilderness!
> America! America!
> God mend thine every flaw,
> Confirm thy soul in self-control,
> Thy liberty in law!

Today I ask that I will look beyond the packaging and not take things at their face value.

July 23rd

On this day in 1745 Charles Stuart (the Young Pretender) landed on Eriskay in the Hebrides. He came with a dozen supporters to begin his bid for the thrones of England and Scotland. Though only 24 when he arrived, Charles quickly gained wide support in the Highlands before entering Edinburgh in September with over two thousand men. Winning the battle of Prestonpans he marched south, reaching Derby before being forced to retreat. The crushing defeat of his forces at Culloden the following April finished the Jacobite rebellion but Charles' subsequent escape and successful eluding of his English pursuers over the ensuing five months ensured that he became a romantic hero.

After the debacle of the 'forty-five' the Hanoverian government pursued a ruthless policy of attrition against Jacobite supporters and the wearing of tartan and the kilt were banned until 1782. Charles died in Rome in 1788, a sad and drunken old man who never managed to make a comeback.
Today's song is a plaintive Jacobite refrain of regret, written probably 30 years after 1745:

> *Bonnie Charlie's now awa'*
> *Safely owre the friendly main;*
> *Mony a heart will break in twa,*
> *Should he ne'er come back again.*
> *English bribes were aa in vain,*
> *An e'en tho puirer we may be;*
> *Siller canna buy the heart*
> *That beats aye for thine and thee*
> *Sweet's the laverock's note and lang,*
> *Lilting wildly up the glen;*
> *But aye to me he sings ae sang,*
> *Will ye no come back again?*

Today I will remember: it is better to try and fail, than not to try at all.

July 24th

On this day in 1802 the great French novelist Alexandre Dumas was born. His thrilling historical novels, such as *The Three Musketeers* and *The Count of Monte Christo* made him famous and rich at the time, although in later life he was forced to flee France to escape his creditors because of his lavish lifestyle.

Dumas was dark-skinned and of mixed race, his grandmother having been a Haitian slave. In spite of this background, Dumas' father had served in the army of Napoleon Bonaparte and risen to the rank of General, an astonishing feat. Dumas worshipped his father who, during his life, had had to endure many insults because of his race.

This is perhaps why D'Artagnan's father, in *The Three Musketeers*, tells his son: "Never submit quietly to the slightest indignity" and why novels by Dumas contain so many heroes who overcome impossible odds and will never allow an insult to go unchallenged.

Today's poem is from *Fantasia* by GK Chesterton:

> Is there not pardon for the brave
> And broad release above,
> Who lost their heads for liberty
> Or lost their hearts for love?
> Or is the wise man wise indeed
> Whom larger thoughts keep whole?
> Who sees life equal like a chart,
> Made strong to play the saner part,
> And keep his head and keep his heart,
> And only lose his soul.

Today I ask that I will keep my personal boundaries strong and not submit quietly to any indignity.

July 25th

On this day on 1909 the French aviator Louis Blériot became the first person to fly an aeroplane across the English Channel. The flight took 36 minutes and terminated in a crash landing near Dover Castle, partly because Blériot had omitted to select a suitable landing site in advance. Blériot successfully claimed the one thousand pounds prize offered by the *Daily Mail* for his feat.

Aviation was a new and dangerous activity at the time and participants such as Bleriot and the Wright brothers had many life-threatening crashes. But thanks partly to their bravery, aviation grew and improved rapidly. When Lindbergh flew the Atlantic for the first time in 1927, Blériot was there to welcome him at Le Bourget. He did not live to see the first commercial transatlantic flight in 1939, but he certainly predicted that it would happen. He died in 1936, a true pioneer.

Today's poem, by Sara Teasdale is named, appropriately, *The Flight*:

> *Look back with longing eyes and know that I will follow,*
> *Lift me up in your love as a light wind lifts a swallow,*
> *Let our flight be far in sun or blowing rain –*
> *But what if I heard my first love calling me again?*
>
> *Hold me on your heart as the brave sea holds the foam,*
> *Take me far away to the hills that hide your home;*
> *Peace shall thatch the roof and love shall latch the door –*
> *But what if I heard my first love calling me once more?*

Today I give thanks for all those pioneers who have pushed forward the frontiers of human knowledge and experience.

July 26th

On this day in 1894 Aldous Huxley, writer and thinker, was born. Though known for his experimental taking of psychedelic drugs before that became fashionable, Huxley is foremost remembered as the author of *Brave New World*, the terrifyingly prophetic account of life in the future that he wrote in 1932.

His predictions of genetically modified babies, boundless consumption, casual sex and drugs seem to get more and more akin to present day life. But Huxley was also deeply spiritual and spent much of his later years researching mysticism and parapsychology.

He probably knew and appreciated this poem, by Edgar Allen Poe, *Alone*:

> *From childhood's hour I have not been*
> *As others were; I have not seen*
> *As others saw; I could not bring*
> *My passions from a common spring.*
> *Then – in my childhood, in the dawn*
> *Of a most stormy life– was drawn*
> *From every depth of good and ill*
> *The mystery which binds me still:*
> *From the torrent, or the fountain,*
> *From the red cliff of the mountain,*
> *From the sun that round me rolled*
> *In its autumn tint of gold,*
> *From the lightning in the sky*
> *As it passed me flying by,*
> *From the thunder and the storm,*
> *And the cloud that took the form*
> *(When the rest of Heaven was blue)*
> *Of a demon in my view.*

Today I ask that I will learn to progress in goodness and spirituality.

July 27th

On this day in 1586 Sir Walter Raleigh introduced tobacco to England. Following Columbus' trip to the New World in 1492, tobacco was soon being described in contemporary accounts:

"men with half-burned wood in their hands and certain herbs to take their smokes, which are some dry herbs put in a certain leaf, also dry, like those the boys make on the day of the Passover of the Holy Ghost; and having lighted one part of it, by the other they suck, absorb, or receive that smoke inside with the breath, by which they become benumbed and almost drunk, and so it is said they do not feel fatigue. These, muskets as we will call them, they call tabacos".

Clearly nicotine has always been addictive and ceasing to smoke will always be hard:

> *It wasn't the whiskey it wasn't the wine*
> *That made such a wreck of this body of mine.*
> *I'll give up the habit I'll manage it yet*
> *When I've had just one last cigarette.*
>
> (Popular song)

Today's poem was written by Raleigh as his epitaph. We assume that he was a smoker himself:

> *Even such is time, which takes in trust*
> *Our youth, our joys, and all we have,*
> *And pays us but with age and dust,*
> *Who in the dark and silent grave*
> *When we have wandered all our ways*
> *Shuts up the story of our days,*
> *And from which earth, and grave, and dust*
> *The Lord will raise me up, I trust.*

Today I ask that I may live free from all addictions.

July 28th

On this day in 1794 Maximilien Robespierre and 22 other revolutionary leaders were guillotined in Paris. The reign of terror was the bloodiest period of the French Revolution. On 5th February 1794, Robespierre stated, succinctly, that "Terror is nothing else than justice, prompt, severe, inflexible." Less than six months later, he experienced it himself.

Today's quote is an account of that very moment, in the inimitable writing of Thomas Carlyle whose *History of the French Revolution* is still a definitive work: "All eyes are on Robespierre's Tumbril, where he, his jaw bound in dirty linen, with his half-dead brother and half-dead Henriot, lie shattered, their 'seventeen hours' of agony about to end. The Gendarmes point their swords at him, to show the people which is he. A woman springs on the Tumbril; clutching the side of it with one hand, waving the other Sibyl-like; and exclaims: 'The death of thee gladdens my very heart, je m'enivre de joi'; Robespierre opened his eyes; 'Scélérat, go down to Hell, with the curses of all wives and mothers!' – At the foot of the scaffold, they stretched him on the ground till his turn came. Lifted aloft, his eyes again opened; caught the bloody axe. Sanson (the executioner) wrenched the coat off him; wrenched the dirty linen from his jaw: the jaw fell powerless, there burst from him a cry; hideous to hear and see. Sanson, thou canst not be too quick!" It minds one of the ditty:

> *The bells of Hell go*
> *Ting a ling a ling*
> *For you but not for me.*
> *O Death where is thy*
> *Sting a ling a ling*
> *O Grave thy mystery?*

Today I ask that I will live my life with kindness and respect and without earning the hatred of others.

July 29th

On this day in 1883 Benito Mussolini was born. He allied Italy with Nazi Germany and Japan in World War Two. Unlike Hitler, he was not good at putting his plans into fruition. He failed to make Italy a powerhouse of economic production as Germany was, and his military campaigns often ended in disaster. History has been kinder to him than to Hitler but, nevertheless, both men were monstrous dictators and each came to a sticky end.

Today's poem is by William Butler Yeats, *The Second Coming*:

> Turning and turning in the widening gyre
> The falcon cannot hear the falconer;
> Things fall apart; the centre cannot hold;
> Mere anarchy is loosed upon the world,
> The blood-dimmed tide is loosed, and everywhere
> The ceremony of innocence is drowned;
> The best lack all conviction, while the worst
> Are full of passionate intensity.
> Surely some revelation is at hand;
> Surely the Second Coming is at hand.
> The Second Coming! Hardly are those words out
> When a vast image out of Spiritus Mundi
> Troubles my sight: a waste of desert sand;
> A shape with lion body and the head of a man,
> A gaze blank and pitiless as the sun,
> Is moving its slow thighs, while all about it
> Wind shadows of the indignant desert birds.
> The darkness drops again but now I know
> That twenty centuries of stony sleep
> Were vexed to nightmare by a rocking cradle,
> And what rough beast, its hour come round at last,
> Slouches towards Bethlehem to be born?

Today I ask that we may all live free of dictatorship.

July 30th

On this day in 1918 the young American poet and soldier Joyce Kilmer was killed in France by a sniper's bullet, just a few weeks before the end of the First World War.

Born into a good middle-class family (his father invented Johnson's baby powder), Kilmer was a devout Catholic and a prolific writer and lecturer comparable to his English contemporaries Belloc and Chesterton. He is chiefly remembered for the simplicity of his writing and his love of nature.

This is exemplified in his best known poem, Trees:

> I think that I shall never see
> A poem lovely as a tree.
> A tree whose hungry mouth is prest
> Against the earth's sweet flowing breast;
> A tree that looks at God all day,
> And lifts her leafy arms to pray;
> A tree that may in summer wear
> A nest of robins in her hair;
> Upon whose bosom snow has lain;
> Who intimately lives with rain.
> Poems are made by fools like me,
> But only God can make a tree.

The poem has been much parodied since it was written in 1913 but its honest simplicity shines through.

Today I ask that I shall appreciate nature in my life.

July 31st

O n this day in 1703 the novelist and pamphleteer Daniel Defoe was placed in a pillory for the crime of seditious libel after publishing a politically satirical pamphlet, and was pelted with flowers.

Defoe is best remembered for his book *Robinson Crusoe* which in 2013 was voted number two in the list of best novels written in English, by the *Guardian* newspaper. It is easy to see why. Supposedly based on a true story, the hero and his sidekick overcome terrible problems to survive on a desert island until they are rescued.

Written over three hundred years ago, when the novel was a virtually unknown genre, its characterisation, pace and structure are masterly. Here is a poem about a different kind of castaway, an old diary. It is by Victorian Poet Augusta Davies Webster, *A Castaway*:

> Poor little diary, with its simple thoughts,
> Its good resolves, its "Studied French an hour,"
> "Read Modern History," "Trimmed up my grey hat,"
> "Darned stockings," "Tatted," "Practised my new song,"
> "Went to the daily service," "Took Bess soup,"
> "Went out to tea." Poor simple diary!
> and did I write it? Was I this good girl?
> ...New clothes to make, then go and say my prayers,
> Or carry soup, or take a little walk
> And pick the ragged-robins in the hedge?
> Then for ambition, (was there ever life
> That could forego that?) To improve my mind
> And know French better and sing harder songs;
> For gaiety, to go, in my best white
> Well washed and starched and freshened with new bows,
> And take tea out to meet the clergyman

Today I ask that I will be thankful for what I have and not envious for what I have not.

August 1st

On this day in 1834, slavery was abolished in the British Empire. In a remarkable turnaround England, the country responsible for transporting an estimated three million Africans to bondage in the Americas, became one of the first in the world to abolish the practice.

Although economic considerations played a part, it was nevertheless a triumph for compassionate humanitarianism and an example of how a long fought campaign can prevail when enough right-minded people are prepared to take action.

John Newton was a slave trader for much of his life but later had a dramatic spiritual awakening and became a clergyman and an abolitionist.

This is the famous hymn that he wrote in 1779:

Amazing Grace, how sweet the sound,
That saved a wretch like me.
I once was lost but now am found,
Was blind, but now I see.
T'was Grace that taught my heart to fear.
And Grace, my fears relieved.
How precious did that Grace appear
The hour I first believed.
Through many dangers, toils and snares
I have already come;
'Tis Grace that brought me safe thus far
And Grace will lead me home.
The Lord has promised good to me.
His word my hope secures.
He will my shield and portion be,
As long as life endures.

Today I ask for the Grace to keep striving to change for the better and never to give up.

August 2nd

On this day in 1865, the Reverend Charles Dodgson (Lewis Carroll), published *Alice's Adventures in Wonderland*. One of the best-loved and most influential books ever published, the story was originally devised as a whimsical fantasy to entertain a group of three children on a boat trip.

Dodgson was also a brilliant mathematician, though he appears to have had difficulty relating to adults. His preference for the company of young girls raised eyebrows at the time but seems to have been innocent.

He wrote this poem years later, about the famous boat trip, *A Boat Beneath a Sunny Sky*:

> *A boat beneath a sunny sky,*
> *Lingering onward dreamily*
> *In an evening of July –*
> *Children three that nestle near,*
> *Eager eye and willing ear,*
> *Pleased a simple tale to hear*
> *Long has paled that sunny sky:*
> *Echoes fade and memories die:*
> *Autumn frosts have slain July.*
> *Still she haunts me, phantomwise,*
> *Alice moving under skies*
> *Never seen by waking eyes.*
> *Children yet, the tale to hear,*
> *Eager eye and willing ear,*
> *Lovingly shall nestle near.*
> *In a Wonderland they lie,*
> *Dreaming as the days go by,*
> *Dreaming as the summers die:*
> *Ever drifting down the stream*
> *Lingering in the golden dream*
> *Life, what is it but a dream?*

Today I ask that I will never lose my curiosity for the wonders in life.

August 3rd

On this day in 1347 six burghers of the besieged French city of Calais surrendered themselves for execution to King Edward III of England, in the hope of relieving the siege. Eustache de Saint Pierre volunteered first, and five other townspeople joined him, ready to face death for the sake of their fellow citizens.

Happily, their lives were spared by the intervention of England's queen, Philippa of Hainault, who persuaded her husband to exercise mercy. Self-sacrifice to the extent of dying in place of another person was held to be one of the finest human acts possible.

Today's poem by Australian Henry Lawson, is about that:

> *Once on a time there lived a man,*
> *But he has lived alway,*
> *And that gaunt, Good Samaritan*
> *Is with us here to-day;*
> *He passes through the city streets*
> *Unnoticed and unknown,*
> *He helps the sinner that he meets –*
> *His sorrows are his own.*
> *He shares his tucker on the track*
> *When things are at their worst*
> *(And often shouts in bars outback*
> *For souls that are athirst).*
> *To-day I see him staggering down*
> *The blazing water-course,*
> *And making for the distant town*
> *With a sick man on his horse.*

Today I ask for the opportunity to work on my selfishness and to help others in need.

August 4th

On this day in 1914, Britain declared war on Germany and so began what is known by many as the Great War. An estimated 16 million people died before the war finished.

Albert Camus, the Algerian French agnostic thinker and philosopher, wrote "In the midst of winter, I found there was, within me, an invincible summer. And that makes me happy. For it says that no matter how hard the world pushes against me, within me, there's something stronger – something better, pushing right back." (From L'Étranger 1942).

Another Frenchman, Jean Paul Sartre, writing somewhat earlier, put it more succinctly: "life begins on the other side of despair" (from La Nausée 1938). Both Camus and Sartre are linked to Existentialism (though Camus rejected this, preferring the word 'Absurdism').

This philosophy proposes that the individual is solely responsible for giving meaning to life and living it passionately and sincerely. Some are guided by a God of their understanding and others follow agnostic, humanist or existentialist paths, but life should be lived as well as possible, even when it appears to have no meaning.

George Herbert says this in his poem, *The Flower*:

> *Who would have thought my shrivelled heart*
> *Could have recovered greenness? It was gone*
> *Quite underground; as flowers depart*
> *To see their mother-root, when they have blown,*
> *Where they together*
> *All the hard weather,*
> *Dead to the world, keep house unknown.*

I ask that today I will do my best in everything and that every choice I make today will be the right one for me and for the rest of mankind.

August 5th

On this day in 1963, the United States, Britain and the Soviet Union signed a treaty in Moscow banning nuclear tests in the atmosphere, space and underwater. Although a very important event at the time, it did not stop a number of other nations, including some very aggressive ones, from developing nuclear weapons.

We live in an imperfect world and we must make the best of it. Setbacks happen often and great achievements take time which is why faith and hope are so important. We must never cease to believe that the power for good that exists in the world is far stronger than the power for evil.

Reinhold Niebuhr said "Nothing that is worth doing can be achieved in our lifetime; therefore we must be saved by hope." We should never cease to hope, however black the world may seem.

Today's poem is by Emily Dickinson, the strange and reclusive New Englander, who died in 1886 and is now considered one of the greatest American poets:

> "Hope" is the thing with feathers
> That perches in the soul
> And sings the tune without the words
> And never stops at all,
> And sweetest in the gale is heard;
> And sore must be the storm
> That could abash the little bird
> That kept so many warm.
> I've heard it in the chillest land
> And on the strangest sea,
> Yet never, in extremity,
> It asked a crumb of me.

I ask today that I will never lose hope. I pray that my faith in the essential power for good in the world will grow stronger.

August 6th

On this day in 1808 English Poet Alfred Lord Tennyson was born. The son of a Lincolnshire clergyman, he held the post of Poet Laureate for a remarkable 42 years and wrote an enormous number of poems.

Considered by many to be the greatest of the Victorian poets, his work has been admired by many for its command of language. Much of his poetry is tinged with sadness and regret, perhaps a result of his father's alcoholism and his own dysfunctional childhood.

The English poet WH Auden unkindly commented: "There was little about melancholia he didn't know; there was little else that he did."

This extract from his poem *Idylls of the King*, on the passing of King Arthur, rather illustrates the point;

And slowly answer'd Arthur from the barge:

"The old order changeth, yielding place to new,
And God fulfils himself in many ways,
Lest one good custom should corrupt the world.
Comfort thyself: what comfort is in me?
I have liv'd my life, and that which I have done
May He within himself make pure! but thou,
If thou shouldst never see my face again,
Pray for my soul. More things are wrought by prayer
Than this world dreams of. Wherefore, let thy voice
Rise like a fountain for me night and day.
For what are men better than sheep or goats
That nourish a blind life within the brain,
If, knowing God, they lift not hands of prayer
Both for themselves and those who call them friend?

Today I ask that every choice I make will be for the right reason and that my conscience will not allow me to get away with falsehood.

August 7th

On this day in 1944 the early computer, Harvard Mark-1, was completed. Built by IBM, it was a room-sized calculator. The machine had a 50 foot long camshaft that synchronised thousands of component parts. This was to lead to the computer revolution that we know today with devices that get smaller and smaller. We can't turn the clock back and ignore new technology, as the 19th century Luddites tried to do by destroying machinery in the Victorian mills of Lancashire and Yorkshire. Learning to accept change is difficult but we have to adapt ourselves. Life, after all, is a continuous process of change that never stops and continues even after we die. Thomas Hardy said so in his poem *Transformations*:

> Portion of this yew
> Is a man my grandsire knew,
> Bosomed here at its foot:
> This branch may be his wife,
> A ruddy human life
> Now turned to a green shoot.
> These grasses must be made
> Of her who often prayed,
> Last century, for repose;
> And the fair girl long ago
> Whom I often tried to know
> May be entering this rose.
> So, they are not underground,
> But as nerves and veins abound
> In the growths of upper air,
> And they feel the sun and rain,
> And the energy again
> That made them what they were!

Today I ask: God grant me the serenity to accept the things I cannot change, courage to change the things I can, and the wisdom to know the difference.

August 8th

On this day in 1864 the founding charter of the International Red Cross and Red Crescent movement was formally adopted in Geneva. We are lucky indeed to live in a world where some people are prepared to help others on an altruistic basis. The Red Cross is a shining example of this, and others spring to mind such as Médecins Sans Frontières and Alcoholics Anonymous. How many lives have been saved by these organisations is hard to tell but it must run into millions. Yet sometimes we take them for granted.

Today's poem is one of the finest ever written on the theme of hope and renewal – a new morning always waits on the far side of night– *God's Grandeur* by Gerard Manley Hopkins:

The world is charged with the grandeur of God.
It will flame out, like shining from shook foil;
It gathers to a greatness, like the ooze of oil
Crushed. Why do men then now not reck his rod?
Generations have trod, have trod, have trod;
And all is seared with trade; bleared, smeared with toil;
And wears man's smudge and shares man's smell: the soil
Is bare now, nor can foot feel, being shod.
And for all this, nature is never spent;
There lives the dearest freshness deep down things;
And though the last lights off the black West went
Oh, morning, at the brown brink eastward, springs –
Because the Holy Ghost over the bent
World broods with warm breast and with ah! Bright wings.

Today I ask that I will be grateful for the unselfish help that I receive in so many ways.

August 9th

On this day in 1922 Philip Larkin, poet, writer and librarian was born. Dubbed 'the poet of low expectations' he once said that deprivation was to him what daffodils were to Wordsworth. His poetry has great humour though often downbeat in content.

He worked most of his life in the university library in Hull, but discontent with his lot was expressed in many of his poems. Larkin was a very English poet in content and outlook, who once said: "I wouldn't mind going to China if I could come back the same day".

AE Housman was another very English poet and this one of his has a flavour of Larkin, *From the Wash*:

> *From the wash the laundress sends*
> *My collars home with ravelled ends:*
> *I must fit, now these are frayed,*
> *My neck with new ones London-made.*
>
> *Homespun collars, homespun hearts,*
> *Wear to rags in foreign parts.*
> *Mine at least's as good as done,*
> *And I must get a London one.*

This poem of Thomas Hardy is equally Larkin-like, to me:

> *I'm Smith of Stoke aged sixty-odd,*
> *I've lived without a dame*
> *From youth-time on; and would to God*
> *My dad had done the same.*

Today I ask that I may be content with my lot and do my daily work as best I can even if it seems boring and repetitive.

August 10th

On this day in 1787, Mozart completed his *Eine Kleine Nachtmusik*, one of his most delightful pieces. By its tone, it must have been written when the composer was in a happy frame of mind. Other works around the same time, *The Marriage of Figaro* and *Don Giovanni*, confirm this same light-hearted feeling.

Four years later, he contracted his final illness and died penniless and was buried in a pauper's grave. Perhaps less well known is his love of schoolboy lavatory humour which marked much of his correspondence.

Here is a translated letter to his much loved cousin Maria after a visit in 1777: "Dearest cozz buzz! I have received reprieved your highly esteemed writing biting...you command that I, too, should could send you my Portrait. Eh bien, I shall mail fail it for sure. Oui, by the love of my skin, I shit on your nose, so it runs down your chin."

I love it – it makes him human. He sent this poem to his mother:

> *Oh mother of mine!*
> *Butter is fine.*
> *Praise and thanks be to Him,*
> *We're alive and full of vim.*
> *Through the world we dash,*
> *Though we're rather short of cash,*
> *But we don't find this provoking*
> *And none of us are choking*
> *At night of farts there is no lack,*
> *Which let off, forsooth, with a powerful crack*

Today I ask that I will love my fellow men and women for what they are and not seek to put them on a pedestal.

August 11th

On this day in 480 BC the Battle of Thermopylae took place. In this narrow pass some 50 miles north of Athens, a small force of seven thousand Greeks held back the invading Persian army of 150,000 for two days. Helped by the nature of the land, the Greeks were doing well and the Persians could make no headway until the traitor, Ephialtes, showed them a secret way round the pass.

Hearing that they had been betrayed and were being outflanked, the Spartan King Leonidas sent his main Greek force south to the safety of the Isthmus of Corinth and remained to fight a rear-guard action with three hundred Spartans and a few hundred others. All were eventually killed. The Spartans were all buried at Thermopylae and the poet Simonides composed this epitaph, famous for its pathos and simplicity: 'O stranger, go tell the Spartans that here we lie, obedient to their commands.' Today's poem is by CP Cavafy:

> Honor to those who in the life they lead
> define and guard a Thermopylae.
> Never betraying what is right,
> consistent and just in all they do
> but showing pity also, and compassion;
> generous when they are rich, and when they are poor,
> still generous in small ways,
> still helping as much as they can;
> always speaking the truth,
> yet without hating those who lie.
> And even more honor is due to them
> when they foresee (as many do foresee)
> that in the end Ephialtis will make his appearance,
> that the Medes will break through after all.

Today I ask that I will not be found wanting in times of need and that I will strive to do my best each day.

August 12th

On this day in 1908 Henry Ford introduced the Model T Ford, the first mass produced car. It went on to sell over 15 million. Ford was able to achieve this by developing his car assembly line through mass production, the first significant industrialist to do so.

Brought up on a farm, Henry Ford got the idea for an assembly line for cars by observing the meat packing industry. Before the Model T, machines such as farm machines, were built individually.

Industrialisation can have negative as well as positive effects on life. Almost one hundred years before the Model T was produced, the English poet William Blake was expressing his concerns in this famous poem:

> And did those feet in ancient time
> Walk upon England's mountains green:
> And was the holy Lamb of God,
> On England's pleasant pastures seen!
> And did the Countenance Divine,
> Shine forth upon our clouded hills?
> And was Jerusalem builded here,
> Among these dark Satanic Mills?
> Bring me my Bow of burning gold;
> Bring me my Arrows of desire:
> Bring me my Spear: O clouds unfold!
> Bring me my Chariot of fire!
> I will not cease from Mental Fight,
> Nor shall my Sword sleep in my hand:
> Till we have built Jerusalem,
> In England's green & pleasant Land.

Today I will strive to understand, rather than to fear change.

August 13th

On this day in 1907, the first motorised taxicab was licensed in New York City. It is strange to think that those familiar yellow cabs have only been around for about one hundred years.

I can't consider this without remembering Joni Mitchell's wonderful 1960s song *Big Yellow Taxi* with its highly relevant messages of caution: "They paved paradise and put up a parking lot."

This is what she said about writing the song: 'I wrote *Big Yellow Taxi* on my first trip to Hawaii. I took a taxi to the hotel and when I woke up the next morning, I threw back the curtains and saw these beautiful green mountains in the distance. Then, I looked down and there was a parking lot as far as the eye could see, and it broke my heart . . . this blight on paradise. That's when I sat down and wrote the song.'

Here is American poet Amy Lowell's poem, *The Taxi*:

> When I go away from you
> The world beats dead
> Like a slackened drum.
> I call out for you against the jutted stars
> And shout into the ridges of the wind.
> Streets coming fast,
> One after the other,
> Wedge you away from me,
> And the lamps of the city prick my eyes
> So that I can no longer see your face.
> Why should I leave you,
> To wound myself upon the sharp edges of the night?

Today I ask that I will appreciate what I have before it's too late.

August 14th

On this day in 1945 Japan surrendered unconditionally to end the Second World War in the Far East. When news of the Japanese surrender broke, Americans spontaneously began celebrating "as if joy had been rationed and saved up", as Life magazine later reported.

In Washington, D.C. a crowd attempted to break into the White House grounds. In Okinawa six people were killed and dozens wounded, as celebrating American soldiers fired guns of all kinds into the sky.

Some Japanese soldiers continued to fight on isolated Pacific islands until at least the 1970s, with the last known Japanese soldier surrendering in 1974.

Here is Wilfred Owen's unforgettable poem *Anthem For Doomed Youth*; though written about another war in another place, it remains one of the most chilling anti-war poems ever written:

> *What passing-bells for these who die as cattle?*
> *Only the monstrous anger of the guns.*
> *Only the stuttering rifles' rapid rattle*
> *Can patter out their hasty orisons.*
> *No mockeries now for them; no prayers nor bells;*
> *Nor any voice of mourning save the choirs, –*
> *The shrill, demented choirs of wailing shells;*
> *And bugles calling for them from sad shires.*
> *What candles may be held to speed them all?*
> *Not in the hands of boys but in their eyes*
> *Shall shine the holy glimmers of goodbyes.*
> *The pallor of girls' brows shall be their pall;*
> *Their flowers the tenderness of patient minds,*
> *And each slow dusk a drawing-down of blinds.*

Today I ask that the world will one day be free of the horrors of war.

August 15th

On this day in 1939 the film *Wizard of Oz* premiered at Grauman's Chinese Theatre, Hollywood. Millions of us love this movie and have our favourite moments, quotes and characters. My own favourite quote is from Dorothy: "Toto, I've a feeling we're not in Kansas anymore."

Judy Garland, who played Dorothy, fell in love with Toto during filming (Toto was female) and wanted to keep her but the owner refused. Toto had her leg broken when someone trod on her during filming – it wasn't all rainbow-land.

In later life, Judy Garland experienced a lot of unhappiness, mainly as a result of failed love affairs. She died from an alcohol and drug induced overdose aged 47 – a tragic end for the girl who, when playing Dorothy, was looking for: "someplace where there isn't any trouble – do you suppose there is such a place, Toto? There must be. It's not a place you can get to by a boat or train. It's far, far away . . . behind the moon . . . beyond the rainbow."

Here is William Wordsworth's poem *The Rainbow*:

> *My heart leaps up when I behold*
> *A rainbow in the sky:*
> *So was it when my life began;*
> *So is it now I am a man;*
> *So be it when I shall grow old,*
> *   Or let me die!*
> *The Child is father of the Man;*
> *I could wish my days to be*
> *Bound each to each by natural piety.*

Today I will remember that regrettably, our dreams may not always come true.

August 16th

On this day in 1819 at St Peter's Field in Manchester, a British cavalry regiment charged into a political gathering, killing 15 people and injuring over four hundred. This was dubbed the Peterloo Massacre, in contemptuous comparison to the Battle of Waterloo five years before.

An eyewitness to the massacre wrote: "Within ten minutes the crowd had been dispersed, at the cost of 11 dead and many injured. Only the wounded, their helpers, and the dead were left behind. For some time afterwards there was rioting in the streets."

Here is an extract from *The Masque of Anarchy*, the poem that Shelley wrote on hearing about Peterloo. It is perhaps the first modern statement of the principle of non-violent resistance:

> *Stand ye calm and resolute,*
> *Like a forest close and mute,*
> *With folded arms and looks which are*
> *Weapons of unvanquished war.*
> *And if then the tyrants dare,*
> *Let them ride among you there;*
> *Slash, and stab, and maim and hew;*
> *What they like, that let them do.*
> *With folded arms and steady eyes,*
> *And little fear, and less surprise,*
> *Look upon them as they slay,*
> *Till their rage has died away:*
> *Then they will return with shame,*
> *To the place from which they came,*
> *And the blood thus shed will speak*
> *In hot blushes on their cheek:*
> *Rise, like lions after slumber*
> *In unvanquishable number!*

Today I ask that I will not fear to stand up for what I believe is right.

August 17th

On this day in 1930 Ted Hughes, British Poet Laureate was born. Apart from his poetry, Hughes is mostly famous for his love life. Married to American poet Sylvia Plath for seven years, she committed suicide after he left her for Assia Wevill, whom he later married.

Tragically, Wevill also committed suicide, killing their young child as well. Hughes was devastated and stopped writing for several years. His third marriage in 1970 was successful and he lived quietly for a further 28 years in both Devon and Yorkshire.

Here is a famous poem by George Herbert that has helped many people struggling to recover from devastating tragedies:

> Love bade me welcome; yet my soul drew back,
>   Guilty of dust and sin.
> But quick-eyed Love, observing me grow slack
>   From my first entrance in,
> Drew nearer to me, sweetly questioning
>   If I lack'd anything.
> 'A guest,' I answer'd, 'worthy to be here:'
>   Love said, 'You shall be he.'
> 'I, the unkind, ungrateful? Ah, my dear,
>   I cannot look on Thee.'
> Love took my hand and smiling did reply,
>   'Who made the eyes but I?'
> 'Truth, Lord; but I have marr'd them: let my shame
>   Go where it doth deserve.'
> 'And know you not,' says Love, 'Who bore the blame?'
>   'My dear, then I will serve.'
> 'You must sit down,' says Love, 'and taste my meat.'
>   So I did sit and eat.

Today I ask that I will be able to handle whatever happens in life, however difficult that may be.

August 18th

On this day in 1587 Virginia Dare was born, the first child of English colonial parents to be born in North America. In 1937, a US postage stamp was issued in her honour. She was born in the ill-fated colony of Roanoake, North Carolina, that was founded in 1585 under a charter given to Sir Walter Raleigh by Queen Elizabeth the 1st. The small colony had difficult relations with the local Indians and may have been attacked and annihilated by them. When the governor John White returned from a trip to England for supplies in 1590, he found the place deserted and no clues as to what had happened.

Perhaps the colonists died from disease or else were forced to put themselves under the protection of the local tribes. Stories later emerged of Europeans seen living in tribal villages. The first child born in North America to pilgrims, or religious migrants, was Peregrine White, aboard the Mayflower in harbour in 1620. Hence this well-known ditty:

> *Peregrine White and Virginia Dare*
> *Were the first real Americans*
> *Anywhere.*
> *Others might find it*
> *Strange to come*
> *Over the ocean*
> *To make a home.*
> *England and memory*
> *Left behind –*
> *But Virginia and Peregrine*
> *Didn't mind.*
> *One of them born*
> *On Roanoke,*
> *And the other cradled*
> *In Pilgrim.*

Today I ask help for all young children, wherever they may be born.

August 19th

On this day in 1561 Mary Queen of Scots arrived in Leith to assume the Scottish throne after spending 13 years in France. Mary was ill-served by her advisors and soon alienated the Scottish Protestants, especially the clergy. Then she made the mistake of marrying for love rather than for political advantage.

Her marriage to her cousin, Lord Darnley, soon soured and her later liaisons with her Italian secretary Rizzio, and the Earl of Bothwell, caused great scandal.

Soon she was at war with her own subjects and eventually forced to flee to the protection of Elizabeth in England; a case of 'from the frying pan into the fire'. The story of her long imprisonment and eventual execution at Fotheringhay Castle is a sad one. Mary liked to write poetry and was fluent in French.

Here is a sonnet she wrote during her long imprisonment, *Que suis-je hélas?*

Alas what am I? What use has my life?
I am but a body whose heart's torn away,
A vain shadow, an object of misery
Who has nothing left but death-in-life.
O my enemies, set your envy all aside;
I've no more eagerness for high domain;
I've borne too long the burden of my pain
To see your anger swiftly satisfied.
And you, my friends who have loved me so true,
Remember, lacking health and heart and peace,
There is nothing worthwhile that I can do;
Ask only that my misery should cease
And that, being punished in a world like this,
I have my portion in eternal bliss.

Today I ask help for all those who are in prison, whatever the reason.

August 20th

On this day in 1619 the first black slaves in North America were brought by Dutch colonists to Jamestown, Virginia. Slave labour was to become a basic fact in the Southern states for the next 250 years until it was outlawed by the 13th amendment in 1865.

In total, about 12 million slaves were brought from Africa to the Americas. The great majority of African slaves were transported to sugar colonies in the Caribbean and Brazil. As life expectancy was short their numbers had to be continually replenished. It was much higher in the U.S. and the slave population began to reproduce; enslaved peoples' numbers grew rapidly, reaching 4 million by the 1860 census.

Phillis Wheatley was the first published African-American woman. Born in West Africa in 1753, she was sold into slavery at the age of seven and transported to North America. She was purchased by the Wheatley family of Boston, who taught her to read and write, and encouraged her poetry. She gained emancipation but died aged 31. George Washington liked her poetry.

See what you think – this is the start of her best-known poem:

> *Twas mercy brought me from my Pagan land,*
> *Taught my benighted soul to understand*
> *That there's a God, that there's a Saviour too:*
> *Once I redemption neither sought nor knew.*
> *Some view our sable race with scornful eye,*
> *"Their colour is a diabolic die."*
> *Remember, Christians, Negro's, black as Cain,*
> *May be refin'd, and join th' angelic train.*

Today I ask help for all those suffering as slaves in the world today.

August 21st

On this day in 750 BC the rape of the Sabine women is said to have taken place. According to the Roman historian Livy this happened after the city of Rome had been founded by the first King, Romulus.

The Roman people, who had arrived in Italy from elsewhere in the Mediterranean basin, were keen to establish themselves and propagate their race. But they were short of womenfolk and they looked to a neighbouring tribe, the Sabines, to form an alliance. But the Sabines wanted none of it.

Romulus and his warriors therefore hatched a plan to hold a joint festival with the Sabines and to abduct their womenfolk in the course of it. According to Livy, in the role of an official historian, this was done in quite a gentlemanly way as Romulus spoke to each woman to persuade her of the benefits of becoming a Roman wife.

Not so much a rape as a coercion, he seems to be saying. Certainly the Sabines were at war with Rome not long after, so probably they saw thing differently. The Roman poet Ovid gave a description in his *Ars Amatoria* (*Art of Love*):

> *As before an eagle, even as a young lamb quails at the sight of a wolf, so shuddered the Sabine women when they beheld these fierce warriors making towards them. Every one turned pale, terror spread throughout the throng, but it showed itself in different ways. Some tore their hair; some swooned away; some wept in silence; some called vainly for their mothers; some sobbed aloud; others seemed stupefied with fear; some stood transfixed; others tried to flee. Nevertheless, the Romans carry off the women, sweet booty for their beds, and to many of them, terror lends an added charm.*

Today I seek help for all the victims of rape and domestic abuse throughout the world.

August 22nd

On this day in 1893, the American writer, humourist and civil rights activist Dorothy Parker was born. Famous for her wit and bittersweet observations on life, Dorothy Parker worked on *Vanity Fair* and the *New Yorker* before moving to Hollywood as a screenwriter. Her private life was characterised by a succession of affairs and failed marriages that she often wryly committed to print. In later life she worked tirelessly for a number of causes, including racial understanding. She died in 1967, leaving her estate to Martin Luther King and the National Association for the Advancement of Colored People.

Her suggested epitaph – "Excuse my Dust" – was oddly relevant because her ashes were left in her agent's filing cabinet for 17 years before being given proper burial.

This minstrel song from Gilbert and Sullivan's *The Mikado* gives an idea of her bittersweet life:

> *A wandering minstrel I –*
> *A thing of shreds and patches,*
> *Of ballads, songs and snatches,*
> *And dreamy lullaby!*
> *And dreamy lullaby!*
> *My catalogue is long,*
> *Through every passion ranging,*
> *And to your humours changing*
> *I tune my supple song!*
> *I tune my supple song!*
> *Are you in sentimental mood?*
> *I'll sigh with you, Oh, sorrow!*
> *On maiden's coldness do you brood? I'll do so, too –*
> *Oh, sorrow, sorrow!*

Today I will remember all those who struggle with relationships and affairs of the heart.

August 23rd

On this day in 1305 Sir William Wallace, freedom fighter of Scotland, was executed for high treason in London. Wallace defeated the English army at the Battle of Stirling Bridge in 1297 and was appointed Guardian of Scotland, serving until his defeat at the Battle of Falkirk in July 1298.

He was captured seven years later and King Edward I of England had him hanged, drawn, and quartered. Wallace remains to this day one of Scotland's great heroes, whose melancholic end at the hands of the English seems to have been followed by so many others in the annals of Scottish history.

It says a lot for the Scots that the tale of Wallace is seen as inspirational, as in this well-known poem by Robert Burns: *Scots Wha Hae*:

> *Scots, wha hae wi' Wallace bled,*
> *Scots, wham Bruce has aften led,*
> *Welcome to your gory bed, – Or to victorie. –*
> *Now 's the day, and now's the hour;*
> *See the front o' battle lour;*
> *See approach proud Edward's power, chains and slaverie.*
> *–*
> *Wha will be a traitor-knave?*
> *Wha can fill a cowards' grave?*
> *Wha sae base as be a Slave? – Let him turn and flie. –*
> *Wha for Scotland's king and law,*
> *Freedom's sword will strongly draw,*
> *Free-Man stand, or Free-Man fa' let him follow me.*
> *– Lay the proud Usurpers low!*
> *Tyrants fall in every foe!*
> *Liberty 's in every blow!*
> *Let us Do – or Die!!!*

Today I ask help for all those suffering under the yoke of tyranny – may they have the courage to rebel, like William Wallace.

August 24th

On this day in 1847 Charlotte Brontë completed the manuscript of *Jane Eyre*. The longest lived of the four Brontë siblings who reached adulthood, she died aged only 39.

Less well known is her father, Patrick Brontë, who outlived all his children to die at the ripe old age of 84. Born to a poor family in Ireland, he had changed his name from Brunty, supposedly in honour of Nelson who had been created Duke of Brontë (in Sicily) in 1799. He may have thought Brontë sounded more distinguished (as indeed it does). Would we have thought any different of the 'Brunty sisters'?

Patrick Brontë wrote some poetry himself, though compared to his children's work it was considerably less successful. Perhaps he had read too much Wordsworth.

Here is a fragment, *The Happy Cottagers*:

> One sunny morn of May,
> When dressed in flowery green
> The dewy landscape, charmed
> With Nature's fairest scene,
> In thoughtful mood
> I slowly strayed
> O'er hill and dale,
> Through bush and glade.
> Throughout the cloudless sky
> Of light unsullied blue,
> The larks their matins raised,
> Whilst on my dizzy view,
> Like dusky motes,
> They winged their way
> Till vanished in the blaze of day.

Today I ask that I will be grateful for the entire corpus of English literature without the need to be too judgemental.

August 25th

On this day in 1944 Paris was liberated, following the success of the D day landings. Mercifully, German general Dietrich von Cholitz disobeyed Hitler's orders to destroy France's beautiful capital city. It was not long before Paris was free.

However, neither the Allies nor the Germans saw Paris as being of particular strategic importance. But to the French its liberation was a huge emotional boost.

By the end of the summer the fighting had moved Eastwards as the Allies raced towards Berlin. A day after liberation, General Charles De Gaulle, leader of the Free French Army, walked down the Champs-Élysées to be greeted by rapturous crowds singing the Marseillaise. It was one of the great moments in the liberation of Europe.

Here is part of that amazing anthem, written by army officer Claude-Joseph Rouget de Lisle at the height of the French Revolution in 1792:

> *Allons enfants de la patrie,*
> *Le jour de gloire est arrivé!*
> *Contre nous de la tyrannie*
> *L'etendard sanglant est levé! (bis)*
> *Entendez-vous dans les campagnes,*
> *Refrain: Aux armes, citoyens!*
> *Formez vos bataillons!*
> *Marchons! Marchons!*
> *Qu'un sang impur*
> *Abreuve nos sillons!'*
> *('Arise, children of the fatherland, the day of glory has come! Tyrrany raises its bloody banner against us – do you hear, in the countryside? To arms, citizens! Form your battalions! March, march, let their impure blood run in our tracks!')*

Today I give thanks for France and the French people.

August 26th

On this day in 1880 the surrealist poet and writer Guillaume Apollinaire was born. He is said to have coined the word 'surreal' and liked to experiment with concrete poetry, where the look and typography of the piece becomes part of the effect.

He also wrote and published several pornographic works. One of the most popular figures in the thriving Paris artistic scene of the early 20th century, Apollinaire fought in the First World War where he was wounded. Before he could fully recover, he died in the flu pandemic of 1918.

Here is an example of his surreal poetry, Evening:

> An eagle descends from this sky white with archangels
>> And you sustain me
> Let them tremble a long while all these lamps
>> Pray pray for me
> The city's metallic and it's the only star
>> Drowned in your blue eyes
> When the tramways run spurting pale fire
>> Over the twittering birds
> And all thet trembles in your eyes of my dreams
>> That a lonely man drinks
> Under flames of gas red like a false dawn
>> O clothed your arm is lifted
> See the speaker stick his tongue out at the listeners
>> A phantom has committed suicide
> The apostle of the fig-tree hangs and slowly rots
>> Let us play this love out then to the end
> Bells with clear chimes announce your birth – see
> The streets are garlanded and the palms advance
>> Towards thee.

Today I can enjoy the surreal, but I must keep focused on the realities of life as well.

August 27th

On this day in 479 BC the invasion of Greece by the Persian emperor Xerxes was defeated by the Spartan general Pausanias at the Battle of Plataea. Xerxes liked to be called by his official name – Shayansha – King of Kings, but the proud Greeks preferred 'Xerxes' (pronounced 'Zurkseez') which has a contemptuous ring to it.

Today many centuries later, we can only marvel at the mind-set of the ancient Greeks, who were prepared to fight so positively for their freedom and their democracy. Byron certainly admired the Greeks so much that he eventually died in their service.

He expresses some of these feelings in his poem, *Isles of Greece*:

> *Isles of Greece, the Isles of Greece!*
> *Where burning Sappho loved and sung,*
> *Where grew the arts of War and Peace,*
> *Where Delos rose, and Phœbus sprung!*
> *Eternal summer gilds them yet,*
> *But all, except their Sun, is set.*
> *The Scian and Teian muse,*
> *The Hero's harp, the Lover's lute,*
> *Have found the fame your shores refuse:*
> *Their place of birth alone is mute*
> *To sounds which echo further west*
> *Than your Sires' "Islands of the Blest."*
> *The mountains look on Marathon*
> *And Marathon looks on the sea;*
> *And musing there an hour alone,*
> *I dreamed that Greece might still be free;*
> *For standing on the Persians' grave,*
> *I could not deem myself a slave*

Today I give thanks for the amazing flowering of ancient Greece and for the benefits it gave to the world.

August 28th

O n this day in 1963 Martin Luther King Jr. delivered his speech "I have a dream," addressing a civil rights march at Lincoln Memorial, Washington DC. He will always be known for his role in the advancement of civil rights using non-violent civil disobedience based on his Christian beliefs.

This is what he said that day: "I have a dream that one day this nation will rise up and live out the true meaning of its creed: 'We hold these truths to be self-evident, that all men are created equal.' I have a dream that one day on the red hills of Georgia, the sons of former slaves and the sons of former slave owners will be able to sit down together at the table of brotherhood".

Five years later, King was gunned down by James Earl Ray outside a Memphis motel. But the dream lives on, though the red hills of Georgia have yet to see brotherhood of the kind that he envisaged. I think that Poet John Bunyan would have got on well with King.

Here is one of his poems, *He That is Down Needs Fear No Fall*:

> *He that is down needs fear no fall,*
> *He that is low no pride;*
> *He that is humble ever shall*
> *Have God to be his guide.*
> *I am content with what I have,*
> *Little be it or much;*
> *And, Lord, contentment still I crave*
> *Because Thou savest such.*
> *Fulness to such a burden is*
> *That go in pilgrimage;*
> *Here little and hereafter bliss*
> *Is best from all to age.*

Today I give thanks for the leadership and inspiration of the great men and women who put the good of their country above personal gain.

August 29th

On this day in 1809 the American physician, poet, professor and author Oliver Wendell Holmes was born. A member of the 'Fireside Poets', his peers acclaimed him as one of the best writers of the day.

A Harvard professor, he was also an important medical reformer and delivered many highly popular lectures on the topics of both science and literature. Of his lecturing style it was said: "He enters, and is greeted by a mighty shout and stamp of applause."

The other professors requested that Holmes teach the last of the five morning lectures, because they knew he could hold the students' attention even though they were tired.

Here is part of one of his poems, about a character that you may recognise, *The Moral Bully*:

The moral bully, though he never swears,
Nor kicks intruders down his entry stairs,
Though meekness plants his backward-sloping hat,
And non-resistance ties his white cravat,
Though his black broadcloth glories to be seen
In the same plight with Shylock's gabardine,
Hugs the same passion to his narrow breast
That heaves the cuirass on the trooper's chest,
Hears the same hell-hounds yelling in his rear
That chase from port the maddened buccaneer,
Feels the same comfort while his acrid words
Turn the sweet milk of kindness into curds,
Or with grim logic prove, beyond debate,
That all we love is worthiest of our hate,
As the scarred ruffian of the pirate's deck,
When his long swivel rakes the staggering wreck!

Today I ask that I will not seek moral superiority or seek to hurt others with words.

August 30th

On this day in 1797, the author Mary Wollstonecraft Shelley was born. Mary's mother, Mary Wollstonecraft, was a well-known feminist and reformer. Young Mary is famous for her scandalous affair with the poet Percy Bysshe Shelley (whom she later married).

The story of the summer that they spent together in Switzerland is well known. It was there that she wrote her famous novel Frankenstein, after an evening that the assembled company had spent telling ghost stories.

As Mary later recounted, she had a waking dream where: "I saw the pale student of unhallowed arts kneeling beside the thing he had put together. I saw the hideous phantasm of a man stretched out, and then, on the working of some powerful engine, show signs of life, and stir with an uneasy, half vital motion."

Here is a poem by Mary, about a nicer kind of dream:

> *Oh, come to me in dreams, my love!*
> *I will not ask a dearer bliss;*
> *Come with the starry beams, my love,*
> *And press mine eyelids with thy kiss.*
> *'Twas thus, as ancient fables tell,*
> *Love visited a Grecian maid,*
> *Till she disturbed the sacred spell,*
> *And woke to find her hopes betrayed.*
> *But gentle sleep shall veil my sight,*
> *And Psyche's lamp shall darkling be,*
> *When, in the visions of the night,*
> *Thou dost renew thy vows to me.*
> *Then come to me in dreams, my love,*
> *I will not ask a dearer bliss;*
> *Come with the starry beams, my love,*
> *And press mine eyelids with thy kiss.*

Today I ask that I will recognise my dreams and learn from them.

August 31st

On this day in 1997 Diana, Princess of Wales, died in a car crash in Paris aged 36. It seems hard to recall today the extraordinary expressions of grief that this event created at the time.

This quote from poet Henry van Dyke was read at her funeral: "Time is too slow for those who wait, too swift for those who fear, too long for those who grieve, too short for those who rejoice, but for those who love, time is eternity." She was buried on the family estate on an island in the middle of a lake.

Sir Walter Scott's poem is today's choice, *The Lady of the Lake*:

> At morn the black-cock trims his jetty wing,
>   'T is morning prompts the linnet's blithest lay,
> All Nature's children feel the matin spring
>   Of life reviving, with reviving day;
> And while yon little bark glides down the bay,
>   Wafting the stranger on his way again,
> Morn's genial influence roused a minstrel gray,
>   And sweetly o'er the lake was heard thy strain,
> Mixed with the sounding harp, O white-haired Allan-bane!
>   Then, stranger, go! Good speed the while,
> Nor think again of the lonely isle.
> 'High place to thee in royal court,
>   High place in battled line,
> Good hawk and hound for sylvan sport!
> Where beauty sees the brave resort,
>   The honoured meed be thine!
> True be thy sword, thy friend sincere,
> Thy lady constant, kind, and dear,
> And lost in love's and friendship's smile
> Be memory of the lonely isle!

Today I remember those who die young.

September 1st

O n this day in 1773 Phyllis Wheatley became the first female African born slave to become a published poet. Born in West Africa she was sold into slavery aged seven and named Phyllis, after the ship that took her to America.

Her poetry was praised by George Washington, King George III and Voltaire. Phyllis lived in Boston as a slave of the Wheatley family, who gave her a good education and eventually her freedom. She visited London and married but her life seems to have gone wrong and she died in poverty aged only 31.

Here is one of her poems, *An Hymn to the Morning*:

> *Attend my lays, ye ever honour'd nine,*
> *Assist my labours, and my strains refine;*
> *In smoothest numbers pour the notes along,*
> *For bright Aurora now demands my song.*
> *Aurora hail, and all the thousand dies,*
> *Which deck thy progress through the vaulted skies:*
> *The morn awakes, and wide extends her rays,*
> *On ev'ry leaf the gentle zephyr plays;*
> *Harmonious lays the feather'd race resume,*
> *Dart the bright eye, and shake the painted plume.*
> *Ye shady groves, your verdant gloom display*
> *To shield your poet from the burning day:*
> *Calliope awake the sacred lyre,*
> *While thy fair sisters fan the pleasing fire:*
> *The bow'rs, the gales, the variegated skies*
> *In all their pleasures in my bosom rise.*
> *See in the east th' illustrious king of day!*
> *His rising radiance drives the shades away –*
> *But Oh! I feel his fervid beams too strong,*
> *And scarce begun, concludes th' abortive song.*

Today I give thanks for brave people like Phyllis Wheatley who are not afraid to face new challenges and try new things.

September 2nd

On this day in 1973 the author and academic JRR Tolkien died. For most of his life an Oxford professor specialising in Anglo Saxon literature, Tolkien produced a remarkable oeuvre of fantasy writing about the world of Middle Earth, where Hobbits and Elves grappled with elemental problems in an oddly human manner.

Tolkien is fondly remembered as a kindly and humorous man by all who knew him. Here are the opening verses from Christina Rossetti's *Goblin Market*. Goblins are not Hobbits of course but I'm not sure what the exact difference is.

Morning and evening
Maids heard the goblins cry:
"Come buy our orchard fruits,
Come buy, come buy:
Apples and quinces,
Lemons and oranges,
Plump unpeck'd cherries,
Melons and raspberries,
Bloom-down-cheek'd peaches,
Swart-headed mulberries,
Wild free-born cranberries,
Crab-apples, dewberries,
Pine-apples, blackberries,
Apricots, strawberries; –
All ripe together

In summer weather –
Morns that pass by,
Fair eves that fly;
Come buy, come buy:
Our grapes fresh from the vine,
Pomegranates full and fine,
Dates and sharp bullaces,
Rare pears and greengages,
Damsons and bilberries,
Taste them and try:
Currants and gooseberries,
Bright-fire-like barberries,
Figs to fill your mouth,
Citrons from the South,
Sweet to tongue and sound to eye;
Come buy, come buy.

Today I am grateful for the added dimensions that fantasy brings and for the way that it stretches my power of imagination.

September 3rd

On this day in 1838 Negro slave Frederick Douglass escaped from captivity in Maryland, USA, dressed as a sailor. Douglass was born into slavery and was 20 years old when he escaped the plantation where he had been working.

Settling in Massachussetts he became first a licensed preacher and then an active abolitionist. A powerful orator, he published several books about his experiences as a slave and held many public government offices. A striking looking man, with dark skin and western features, his father was rumoured to be the plantation owner where he had been born.

Douglass married twice, the first to a black woman, the second time to a white woman. He answered the critics by saying that his first marriage had been to someone the colour of his mother, and his second to someone the colour of his father.

Today's poem is about slavery, by Henry Wadsworth Longfellow, *The Slave Singing at Midnight*:

> *Loud he sang the psalm of David!*
> *He, a Negro and enslaved,*
> *Sang of Israel's victory,*
> *Sang of Zion, bright and free.*
> *In that hour, when night is calmest,*
> *Sang he from the Hebrew Psalmist,*
> *In a voice so sweet and clear*
> *That I could not choose but hear,*
> *Songs of triumph, and ascriptions,*
> *Such as reached the swart Egyptians,*
> *When upon the Red Sea coast*
> *Perished Pharaoh and his host. And what*
> *   earthquake's arm of might*
> *Breaks his dungeon-gates at night?*

Today I ask for freedom for all those in the world who are slaves.

September 4th

On this day in 1998 the astronaut John Glenn became the oldest man in space when he orbited the earth at the age of 77. Already a national hero, John Glenn had become the first American in space in 1962 at the start of the space age.

His extraordinary life started much earlier in the US Air Force during World War II when he flew 59 combat missions. Going into politics in later life, he was a US Senator for over 20 years and was still a Senator when he went into space a second time.

This exploit at such an advanced age gave inspiration to millions. The view from a space capsule is said to be truly awesome. Shakespeare never had that experience yet he could write movingly about his own view of the world.

Here is *Sonnet XXXIII*:

> *Full many a glorious morning have I seen*
> *Flatter the mountain tops with sovereign eye,*
> *Kissing with golden face the meadows green,*
> *Gilding pale streams with heavenly alchemy;*
> *Anon permit the basest clouds to ride*
> *With ugly rack on his celestial face,*
> *And from the forlorn world his visage hide,*
> *Stealing unseen to west with this disgrace:*
> *Even so my sun one early morn did shine,*
> *With all triumphant splendour on my brow;*
> *But out, alack, he was but one hour mine,*
> *The region cloud hath mask'd him from me now.*
> *Yet him for this my love no whit disdaineth;*
> *Suns of the world may stain when heaven's sun staineth.*

Today I give thanks for the bravery of men like John Glenn and I welcome the inspiration his achievements bring to all those experiencing old age.

September 5th

On this day in 1661 the French Superintendent of Finance, Nicolas Fouquet was arrested on suspicion of mismanagement of the king's finances. The young King Louis XIV, succeeding at the age of five, had famously said upon coming of age, that he would be 'his own first minister'.

He had distrusted Fouquet for some time but especially after paying a visit to Vaux le Vicomte, the huge château that Fouquet had built and where Louis was entertained to a lavish Fête. A few weeks later Fouquet was arrested, tried and imprisoned in the fortress of Pignerol. The whole affair was an example of the harsh and decisive way in which the young Louis established his authority. Louis had grown up with a deep distrust of the aristocracy and of Paris, after witnessing as a child the revolt of many nobles against the monarchy (known as the 'fronde') which had turned Paris into a battleground for several years. This led to him establishing a new court at Versailles, a village located outside of Paris.

Today's poem by the 18th century poet Isaac Watts, is based on *Psalm 146, Put Not Your Trust in Princes*:

> I'll praise my Maker while I've breath,
> And when my voice is lost in death,
> Praise shall employ my nobler powers;
> My days of praise shall ne'er be past,
> While life, and thought, and being last,
> Or immortality endures.
> Why should I make a man my trust?
> Princes must die and turn to dust;
> Vain is the help of flesh and blood:
> Their breath departs,
> Their pomp, and power,
> And thoughts, all vanish in an hour,
> Nor can they make their promise good

Today I give thanks that I do not rely on the patronage of others for my well-being.

September 6th

On this day in 1860 the first test match in England was played against Australia at the Oval cricket ground. Along with the English language, cricket has been said to be one of the unifying factors of the British Empire.

It remains popular in most of the great nations that were formerly part of the Empire – Australia, New Zealand, India, South Africa and the West Indies. Even in the USA there are cricket clubs.

The game remains an essential part of the British character, as this poem by Sir Henry Newbolt confirms, *Vitae Lampada*:

> There's a breathless hush in the Close to-night –
> Ten to make and the match to win –
> A bumping pitch and a blinding light,
> An hour to play and the last man in.
> And it's not for the sake of a ribboned coat,
> Or the selfish hope of a season's fame,
> But his captain's hand on his shoulder smote
> "Play up! play up! And play the game!"
> The sand of the desert is sodden red, –
> Red with the wreck of a square that broke; –
> The Gatling's jammed and the Colonel dead,
> And the regiment blind with dust and smoke.
> This is the word that year by year,
> While in her place the school is set,
> Every one of her sons must hear,
> And none that hears it dare forget.
> This they all with a joyful mind
> Bear through life like a torch in flame,
> And falling fling to the host behind –
> "Play up! Play up! And play the game!"

Today I give thanks for the strength of the British character.

September 7th

O n this day in 1497 the imposter Perkin Warbeck declared himself King Richard IV and entered Exeter with an army of six thousand men. The English King Henry VII sent an army to confront him and Warbeck duly surrendered. He was taken to the Tower of London but treated well. However, after trying unsuccessfully to escape, he was taken to Tyburn and hanged. Perkin Warbeck had claimed that he was Richard Plantagenet, son of Edward IV, one of the two princes in the tower rumoured to have been murdered by Richard III of ill repute.

Shakespeare put it well – a king can never relax (*Henry the Fourth, Part 2*):

> *How many thousand of my poorest subjects*
> *Are at this hour asleep! O sleep, O gentle sleep,*
> *Nature's soft nurse, how have I frighted thee,*
> *That thou no more wilt weigh my eyelids down*
> *And steep my senses in forgetfulness?*
> *Wilt thou upon the high and giddy mast*
> *Seal up the ship-boy's eyes, and rock his brains*
> *In cradle of the rude imperious surge*
> *And in the visitation of the winds,*
> *Who take the ruffian billows by the top,*
> *Curling their monstrous heads and hanging them*
> *With deafening clamour in the slippery clouds,*
> *That, with the hurly, death itself awakes?*
> *Canst thou, O partial sleep, give thy repose*
> *To the wet sea-boy in an hour so rude,*
> *And in the calmest and most stillest night,*
> *With all appliances and means to boot,*
> *Deny it to a king? Then happy low, lie down!*
> *Uneasy lies the head that wears a crown.*

Today I give thanks for the blessing of untroubled sleep that comes from an easy conscience.

September 8th

On this day in 1886 the English poet Siegfried Sassoon was born. Sassoon was christened Siegfried because his mother loved Wagner's opera. He is chiefly remembered for his poetry of the First World War, such as *The General and Everyone Sang*, which showed pathos, triviality and horror of the times.

Sassoon distinguished himself by several insane sounding acts of bravery such as taking a German trench single handed – then staying there for an hour to read poetry. He won the Military Cross but was later placed in a mental hospital with shell shock where he befriended the poet Wilfred Owen.

Surviving the war, he also wrote novels and biographies including the well-received *Memoirs of a Fox Hunting Man*. He died at the age of 81.

Here is another famous poem, by Rupert Brooke, a casualty in that same war, *A Memory*:

> Somewhile before the dawn I rose, and stept
> Softly along the dim way to your room,
> And found you sleeping in the quiet gloom,
> And holiness about you as you slept.
> I knelt there; till your waking fingers crept
> About my head, and held it. I had rest
> Unhoped this side of Heaven, beneath your breast.
> I knelt a long time, still; nor even wept.
> It was great wrong you did me; and for gain
> Of that poor moment's kindliness, and ease,
> And sleepy mother-comfort! Child, you know
> How easily love leaps out to dreams like these,
> Who has seen them true. And love that's wakened so
> Takes all too long to lay asleep again.

Today I give thanks for the human spirit that can give poetry preference over fighting.

September 9th

On this day in 1087 King William I of England (the Conqueror) died. The Norman Conquest changed Saxon England for ever.

As soon as William breathed his last, at Rouen, the wealthy nobles, including his sons, hurriedly left to protect their estates, after stripping William of his valuables and leaving him virtually naked on the floor. It was left to the local monks to arrange the funeral and burial. His tomb was desecrated in later centuries; an ignoble end for a man who had changed history.

Today's poem by Lord Byron, is on a similar theme *All Is Vanity Saith The Preacher*:

> Fame, wisdom, love, and power were mine,
> And health and youth possess'd me;
> My goblets blush'd from every vine,
> And lovely forms caress'd me;
> I sunn'd my heart in beauty's eyes,
> And felt my soul grow tender;
> All earth can give, or mortal prize,
> Was mine of regal splendour.
> There rose no day, there roll'd no hour
> Of pleasure unembitter'd;
> And not a trapping deck'd my power
> That gall'd not while it glitter'd.
> The serpent of the field, by art
> And spells, is won from harming;
> But that which coils around the heart,
> Oh! Who hath power of charming?
> It will not list to wisdom's lore,
> Nor music's voice can lure it;
> But there it stings for evermore
> The soul that must endure it.

Today I will remember that fame and fortune are temporal.

September 10th

O n this day in 1638 the Infanta Maria Teresa of Spain was born, later to become the wife of Louis XIV of France. Her virtue and piety were legendary and she fulfilled her duty as queen by producing a male heir to the throne.

She is said to have genuinely loved her husband in spite of having to tolerate his many illicit love affairs and the presence of his official mistresses at court.

Maria Teresa and Louis were first cousins and remained friends throughout the marriage until her untimely death at the age of 44. Upon her death, the king said: "This is the first trouble which she has given me."

Today's poem is about love and life, by George Herbert, *The World*:

> *Love built a stately house, where Fortune came,*
> *And spinning fancies, she was heard to say*
> *That her fine cobwebs did support the frame,*
> *Whereas they were supported by the same;*
> *But Wisdom quickly swept them all away.*
> *Reforméd all at length with menaces.*
> *Then entered Sin, and with that sycamore*
> *Whose leaves first sheltered man from drought and dew,*
> *Working and winding slily evermore,*
> *The inward walls and summers cleft and tore;*
> *But Grace shored these, and cut that as it grew.*
> *Then Sin combined with death in a firm band,*
> *To raze the building to the very floor;*
> *Which they effected,*
> *none could them withstand;*
> *But Love and Grace took Glory by the hand,*
> *And built a braver palace than before.*

Today I will give thanks for all the love in the world.

September 11th

On this day in 1885 the English writer, poet and painter DH Lawrence was born into a Nottinghamshire working class family. His powerful writing was often seen as scandalous and overly sensual, particularly regarding sexual imagery.

The notoriety of his writing and painting forced Lawrence to live abroad for the last 12 years of his life. Much scandal was attached to his books both during his life and later; his novel Lady Chatterley's Lover was the subject of a court case in 1960. All this has tended to obscure the fact that he wrote some very fine poetry. Here is an example, *Lightening*:

I felt the lurch and halt of her heart
Next my breast, where my own heart was beating;
And I laughed to feel it plunge and bound,
And strange in my blood-swept ears was the sound
Of the words I kept repeating,
Repeating with tightened arms, and the hot blood's blind-
fold art.
Her breath flew warm against my neck,
Warm as a flame in the close night air;
And the sense of her clinging flesh was sweet
Where her arms and my neck's blood-surge could meet.
Holding her thus, did I care
That the black night hid her from me, blotted out every
speck?
I leaned me forward to find her lips,
And claim her utterly in a kiss,
When the lightning flew across her face,
And I saw her for the flaring space
Almost I hated her, she was so good.
Hated myself, and the place, and my blood,
Which burned with rage, as I bade her come
Home, away home, ere the lightning floated forth again.

Today I ask that I will be true to myself and strive to do my best in all things.

September 12th

On this day in 510 BC the Athenian Army under its clever general Miltiades defeated a much larger Persian Army at the Battle of Marathon. Miltiades had previously served in the Persian army and knew the tactics they used. He ordered the Athenians to attack at a run, not giving the feared Persian bowmen time to get ready. The plan worked and the Persians were driven back into the sea. The Spartans, who arrived too late to help, could not believe the result and insisted on touring the battlefield to count the dead; but the Athenians knew they had been lucky and later put great effort into enlarging their army and their fleet.

Here is a description of a battle from ancient China by the poet Chu Yuan writing in about 300 BC, *Battle*:

> *We grasp our battle-spears: we don our breast-plates of hide.*
> *The axles of our chariots touch: our short swords meet.*
> *Standards obscure the sun: the foe roll up like clouds.*
> *Arrows fall thick: the warriors press forward.*
> *They menace our ranks: they break our line.*
> *The left-hand trace-horse is dead: the one on the right is smitten.*
> *The fallen horses block our wheels: they impede the yoke-horses!*
> *They grasp their jade drum-sticks: they beat the sounding drums.*
> *Heaven decrees their fall: the dread Powers are angry.*
> *The warriors are all dead: they lie on the moor-field.*
> *They issued but shall not enter: they went but shall not return.*
> *The plains are flat and wide: the way home is long.*
> *Their swords lie beside them: their black bows, in their hand.*
> *Though their limbs were torn, their hearts could not be repressed.*
> *They were more than brave: they were inspired with the spirit of*
> *   Wu.*

Today I ask that the world will one day become free of all wars.

September 13th

On this day in AD 122 work began on building Hadrian's Wall across Northern Britain. Hadrian was one of Rome's greatest emperors. During his 21 year reign he visited nearly every province and consolidated the empire, the Wall being one example.

His hard work ensured that the Pax Romana continued for at least another 50 years. Hadrian was essentially a soldier and normally wore military uniform but he was also a cultured and sensitive man.

A longtime lover of Greece and its culture, he is also known for his close relationship with the young Greek Antinous whose death from drowning in the Nile, during a visit to Egypt, is said to have devastated him. He died aged 62 of natural causes, fairly unusual for a Roman emperor.

Here is the well-known poem that he wrote shortly before his death:

> Animula, vagula, blandula
> Hospes comesque corporis
> Quae nunc abibis in loca
> Pallidula, rigida, nudula,
> Nec, ut soles, dabis iocos

This translation is by Marguerite Yourcenar whose scholarly work *Hadrian's Memoirs*, opened the eyes of many to the greatness of the man:

> Little soul, gentle and drifting,
> guest and companion of my body,
> now you will dwell below in pallid places, stark and bare;
> there you will abandon your play of yore.

Today I give thanks for all world leaders who have the humanity and the spirituality to consider their own souls.

September 14th

On this day in 1849 the Russian physiologist Ivan Pavlov was born. During the 1890s Pavlov was looking at salivation in dogs in response to being fed, when he noticed that his dogs would begin to salivate whenever he entered the room, even when he was not bringing them food.

Pavlov's observations led him to formulate his concept of the conditioned (i.e. learned) reflex. In his most famous experiment, he sounded a tone just before presenting dogs with food; from this they were quickly conditioned to begin salivating every time he sounded the tone. This ground-breaking work won him the Nobel Prize in 1904. Pavlov lived through the years of revolution in Russia and died in 1936. The phrase 'Pavlovian reaction' lives on.

Here is a poem about learning, by Alexander Pope, *A Little Learning*:

> *A little learning is a dangerous thing;*
> *Drink deep, or taste not the Pierian Spring:*
> *There shallow draughts intoxicate the brain,*
> *And drinking largely sobers us again.*
> *Fired at first sight with what the Muse imparts,*
> *In fearless youth we tempt the heights of Arts ;*
> *So pleased at first the towering Alps we try,*
> *Mount o'er the vales, and seem to tread the sky;*
> *The eternal snows appear already past,*
> *And the first clouds and mountains seem the last;*
> *But those attained, we tremble to survey*
> *The growing labours of the lengthened way;*
> *The increasing prospect tires our wandering eyes,*
> *Hill peep o'er hills, and Alps on Alps arise!*

Today I ask that I will never cease to learn even little things.

September 15th

On this day in 1889 the American writer and humourist Robert Benchley was born. A founding member of the famous Algonquin Round Table in New York, Benchley wrote prolifically for the New Yorker and Vanity Fair and influenced many writers, especially James Thurber and Dorothy Parker (with whom he shared the telegraphic address 'park bench').

He is not so well known these days but some of his sayings live on, such as: "drawing on my fine command of the English language, I said nothing." His piece 'Kiddie-Kar Travel' which begins "In America there are two classes of travel – first class, and with children," is one of the funniest accounts ever written on travel. Benchley developed an alcohol problem in later life and died of cirrhosis, a sad end for one who gave pleasure to so many.

Here is a surreal poem by another humourist, Edward Lear, *Cold are the Crabs*:

> *Cold are the crabs that crawl on yonder hills,*
> *Colder the cucumbers that grow beneath,*
> *And colder still the brazen chops that wreathe*
> *The tedious gloom of philosophic pills!*
> *For when the tardy film of nectar fills*
> *The simple bowls of demons and of men,*
> *There lurks the feeble mouse, the homely hen,*
> *And there the porcupine with all her quills.*
> *Yet much remains – to weave a solemn strain*
> *That lingering sadly – slowly dies away,*
> *Daily departing with departing day*
> *A pea-green gamut on a distant plain*
> *When wily walruses in congresses meet –*
> *Such, such is life –*

Today I ask that I will never cease to value friendship and that I will work to nurture those that I have.

September 16th

On this day in 1880 the British poet Alfred Noyes was born. A teacher's son from the Midlands, Noyes went to Oxford where his first poems were published. He married the daughter of the American Consul in Hull and, on a trip with her to New England, was offered a job at Princeton University where he became a visiting professor. Among his students was F. Scott Fitzgerald.

His best known poem, *The Highwayman*, is a romantic ballad that begins: "The wind was a torrent of darkness among the gusty trees. The moon was a ghostly galleon tossed upon cloudy seas". One feels that Noyes himself loved to travel.

Here is part of a poem by the American poet Vachel Lindsay, entitled *Traveller Heart*:

> *I would be one with the dark, dark earth: –*
> *Follow the plough with a yokel tread.*
> *I would be part of the Indian corn,*
> *Walking the rows with the plumes o'erhead.*
> *I would be one with the lavish earth,*
> *Eating the bee-stung apples red:*
> *Walking where lambs walk on the hills;*
> *By oak-grove paths to the pools be led.*
> *I would be one with the dark-bright night*
> *When sparkling skies and the lightning wed –*
> *Walking on with the vicious wind*
> *By roads whence even the dogs have fled.*
> *I shall be one with all pit-black things*
> *Finding their lowering threat unsaid:*
> *Stars for my pillow there in the gloom –*
> *Oak-roots arching about my head!*
> *Sweet with the life of my sunburned days*
> *When the sheaves were ripe, and the apples red.*

Today I ask that I will never trivialise the important things in life.

September 17th

On this day in 1923 the American country singer and songwriter Hank Williams was born. He grew up in rural Alabama but moved to Memphis where he worked and performed at the Grand Ole Opry. He produced a large number of hit songs including *Your Cheatin' Heart* and *Hey Good Lookin'*.

However, his lifestyle and addiction to alcohol and prescription drugs took their toll and he died at the early age of 29 from alcohol related problems. Most people who heard him sing did not forget the emotional intensity of the experience.

John Donne, writing three hundred years before Hank Williams, was another who put great emotional intensity into his work, such as this one, *Sacred Sonnet*:

> *Batter my heart, three-person'd God, for you*
> *As yet but knock, breathe, shine, and seek to mend;*
> *That I may rise and stand, o'erthrow me, and bend*
> *Your force to break, blow, burn, and make me new.*
> *I, like an usurp'd town to another due,*
> *Labor to admit you, but oh, to no end;*
> *Reason, your viceroy in me, me should defend,*
> *But is captiv'd, and proves weak or untrue.*
> *Yet dearly I love you, and would be lov'd fain,*
> *But am betroth'd unto your enemy;*
> *Divorce me, untie or break that knot again,*
> *Take me to you, imprison me, for I,*
> *Except you enthrall me, never shall be free,*
> *Nor ever chaste, except you ravish me.*

Today I ask that I will always do my best to help those struggling with addiction problems.

September 18th

On this day in 1846 the poet and writer Robert Browning and the poetess Elizabeth Barrett decided to elope together. Though several years older than Browning, Elizabeth became a loving wife and muse to her husband – some of his work had not been well received.

Soon, however, his work gained more popularity as in his famous *Childe Roland to the Dark Tower Came*:

> *My first thought was, he lied in every word,*
> *That hoary cripple, with malicious eye*
> *Askance to watch the working of his lie*
> *On mine, and mouth scarce able to afford*
> *Suppression of the glee, that pursed and scored*
> *Its edge, at one more victim gained thereby.*

Unlike the narrative tone of Robert's poem, Elizabeth's writing is more expressive of her feelings. This is from *The Soul's Travelling*:

> *God, God! With a child's voice I cry,*
> *Weak, sad, confidingly – God, God!*
> *Thou knowest, eyelids, raised not always up*
> *Unto Thy love (as none of ours are), droop*
> *As ours, o'er many a tear!*
> *Thou knowest, though Thy universe is broad,*
> *Two little tears suffice to cover all:*
> *Thou knowest, Thou, who art so prodigal*
> *Of beauty, we are oft but stricken deer*
> *Expiring in the woods – that care for none*
> *Of those delightsome flowers they die upon.*

Today I reflect on the strength that love can give to two people.

September 19th

On this day in 1911 the English novelist William Golding was born. In 1983 he won the Nobel Prize for Literature. His first and most famous novel is *Lord of the Flies*, which tells the story of a group of schoolboys who are marooned on a desert island and revert to savagery.

It was not published until 1953, when Golding was 42. Golding had a distinguished war record in the navy and afterwards lived quietly in the west of England.

This poem by Robert Browning has some of the feeling of abandonment that the boys in William Golding's famous book must have felt, *Waring*:

> *What's become of Waring*
> *Since he gave us all the slip,*
> *Chose land-travel or seafaring,*
> *Boots and chest, or staff and scrip,*
> *Rather than pace up and down*
> *any longer London-town?*
> *Who'd have guessed it from his lip,*
> *Or his brow's accustomed bearing,*
> *On the night he thus took ship,*
> *Or started landward? – little caring*
> *I left his arm that night myself*
> *For what's-his-name's, the new prose-poet,*
> *That wrote the book there, on the shelf –*
> *How, forsooth, was I to know it*
> *If Waring meant to glide away*
> *Like a ghost at break of day?*
> *Never looked he half so gay!*

Today I ask to be proactive and not allow myself to be driven by events into self-defeating behaviour.

September 20th

On this day in 1863 Jakob Grimm died, the elder of the German brothers Grimm. A notable scholar, his great work was the definitive German Dictionary (Deutsches Wortebuch) which was unfinished at his death. Its 33 volumes were finally completed in 1961.

The Grimm's were among the best-known storytellers of folk tales, and popularised stories such as *Cinderella, The Frog Prince, Hansel and Gretel, Rapunzel, Rumpelstiltskin*, and *Snow White*. Their first collection of folk tales, Children's and Household Tales (Kinder– und Hausmärchen), was published in 1812 and is now world famous.

English fairy tales tend to be a little bit more surreal than the frighteningly realistic German versions, such as in this poem by' Lewis Carroll, *Jabberwocky*:

> *'Twas brillig, and the slithy toves*
> *Did gyre and gimble in the wabe:*
> *All mimsy were the borogoves,*
> *And the mome raths outgrabe.*
> *"Beware the Jabberwock, my son!*
> *The jaws that bite, the claws that catch!*
> *Beware the Jubjub bird, and shun*
> *The frumious Bandersnatch!"*
> *One, two! One, two! And through and through*
> *The vorpal blade went snicker-snack!*
> *He left it dead, and with its head*
> *He went galumphing back.*
> *"And hast thou slain the Jabberwock?*
> *Come to my arms, my beamish boy!*
> *O frabjous day! Callooh! Callay!"*
> *He chortled in his joy*

Today I give thanks for all those adults who can inspire and help children.

September 21st

On this day in 19 BC the Roman poet Virgil (Publius Virgilius Maro) died. A shy and retiring bachelor from northern Italy who was physically too weak to be a soldier, Virgil lived through the civil wars that ended the Roman Republic, the assassination of Julius Caesar and the foundation of the Roman Empire under Augustus, the first emperor.

His most famous work, The Aeneid, traces the foundation of Rome back to the fall of Troy and the subsequent wanderings of its hero, the Trojan Aeneas. It can thus be seen as a work of propaganda designed to glorify and legitimise the newly created Roman Empire. Though modelled on Homer, it is nevertheless a magnificent and poetic work of art in its own right.

Arguably Virgil's finest poetry is contained in the *Eclogues*, a collection of pastoral poems with idyllic themes such as the love of shepherds and shepherdesses which show Virgil's love of the countryside. Legend has it that Saint Paul visited Virgil's tomb in Naples and wept. The *Eclogues* inspired many subsequent poets, not least Shakespeare.

Here is a taste of Virgil from the start of the exquisite *Eclogue VIII*:

> *Saepibus in nostris parvam te roscida mala*
> *(Dux ego vester eram) vidi cum matre legentem.*
> *Alter ab undecimo tum me iam acceperat annus,*
> *Iam fragilis poteram a terra contingere ramos:*
> *Ut vidi, ut perii, ut me malus abstulit error!*
> *'In our orchard I saw you picking dewy apples with your*
> *mother (I was showing you the way). I had just turned*
> *twelve years old, and I could reach the brittle branches even*
> *from the ground: how I watched you! how I fell in love!*
> *How an awful madness swept me away!'*

Today I pray that I will be inspired and grateful for the poetry in the world.

September 22nd

On this day in 1692 the last of a group of 20 people were hanged for witchcraft in Salem, Massachusetts. This event was not unique, but simply an American example of the much broader phenomenon of witch trials from the 15th to 18th centuries.

In 1953 Arthur Miller wrote his famous play *The Crucible* about the Salem trials, while senator Joseph McCarthy was conducting his notorious investigations into 'un-American activities' (i.e. communist sympathies) among well-known personalities such as Orson Welles, Charlie Chaplin and Paul Robeson. Miller himself was questioned by the House of Representatives' Committee on Un-American Activities in 1956 and convicted of "Contempt of Congress" for refusing to identify others present at meetings he had attended.

Today's poem is by Khalil Gibran *On Crime and Punishment*:

Then one of the judges of the city stood forth and said, "Speak to us of Crime and Punishment."
And he answered saying:
It is when your spirit goes wandering upon the wind,
That you, alone and unguarded,
Commit a wrong unto others and therefore unto yourself.
And for that wrong committed must you knock and wait a while unheeded at the gate of the blessed.
Like the ocean is your god-self;
It remains for ever undefiled.
And like the ether it lifts but the winged.
Even like the sun is your god-self;
It knows not the ways of the mole nor seeks it the holes of the serpent.
But your god-self does not dwell alone in your being.

Today I pray for all victims of extremism and intolerance.

September 23rd

On this day in 1215 Kublai Khan, grandson of Genghis Khan was born, soon to be ruler of the vast Mongol Empire in Asia.

Kublai was an enlightened ruler, supporting both the Buddhist and Islam religions. He was also interested in trade; Marco Polo, the Venetian merchant, spent 17 years at his court.

Samuel Taylor Coleridge was in an opium induced trance when he wrote this poem:

In Xanadu did Kubla Khan
A stately pleasure-dome decree
Where Alph, the sacred river, ran
Through caverns measureless to man
  Down to a sunless sea. A damsel with a dulcimer
  In a vision once I saw:
  It was an Abyssinian maid
  And on her dulcimer she played,
  Singing of Mount Abora.
  Could I revive within me
  Her symphony and song,
  To such a deep delight 'twould win me,
That with music loud and long,
I would build that dome in air,
That sunny dome! those caves of ice
And all who heard should see them there,
And all should cry, Beware! Beware!
His flashing eyes, his floating hair!
Weave a circle round him thrice,
And close your eyes with holy dread
For he on honey-dew hath fed,
And drunk the milk of Paradise.

Today I give thanks that I can enjoy the beauty of the Orient without mood altering drugs.

September 24th

On this day in 1897 Annie Kopchovsky arrived back in Boston, Massachusetts to become the first women to cycle round the world. She was a free-thinking young woman, mother of three children, who reinvented herself as the daring "Annie Londonderry" – entrepreneur, athlete and globetrotter.

Travelling with a change of clothes and a pearl-handled revolver, she earned her way by carrying advertising banners through countries around the world. She saw the venture as a test of a woman's ability to fend for herself. Despite having never ridden a bicycle, she began her journey via New York to France and Egypt, then India and points east, returning to the United States at San Francisco. It took her 15 months. She later said "I believe I can do anything that any man can do."

Today's poem is about an Australian cyclist: *Mulga Bill's Bicycle* by A.B. "Banjo" Paterson:

Twas Mulga Bill, from Eaglehawk, that caught the cycling craze;
He turned away the good old horse that served him many days;
He dressed himself in cycling clothes, resplendent to be seen;
He hurried off to town and bought a shining new machine;
And as he wheeled it through the door, with air of lordly pride,
The grinning shop assistant said, "Excuse me, can you ride?"
See here, young man," said Mulga Bill, "from Walgett to the sea,
From Conroy's Gap to Castlereagh, there's none can ride like me.
There's nothing clothed in hair or hide, or built of flesh or steel,
There's nothing walks or jumps, or runs, on axle, hoof, or wheel,
But what I'll sit, while hide will hold and girths and straps are tight:
I'll ride this here two-wheeled concern right straight away at sight."

Today I ask that I will appreciate the freedom to roam that cycling allows me.

September 25th

On this day in 1066 King Harold of England defeated an invading army of Norwegians at Stamford Bridge in Yorkshire. Harald had been at Hastings on the south coast, awaiting an invasion by the Normans from France (it came sure enough a few weeks later). He was forced to march his army up to Yorkshire, a distance of 185 miles, to fight off this new threat.

Three days later, the Normans landed on the south coast and Harald had to rush his exhausted army back again to face them at Hastings. No wonder that the Normans, under William the Conqueror, won the battle. Perhaps Harald had a foreboding about his death.

Today's poem is from Carmina Gadelica, the ancient Celtic poetry of the Highlands and Islands of Scotland, *The Battle to Come*:

> *Jesus, Thou son of Mary, I call on Thy name,*
> *And on the name of John, the apostle beloved,*
> *And on the names of all the saints in the red domain,*
> *To shield me in the battle to come,*
> *To shield me in the battle to come.*
> *When the mouth shall be closed,*
> *When the eye shall be shut,*
> *When the breath shall cease to rattle,*
> *When the heart shall cease to throb,*
> *When the heart shall cease to throb.*
> *When the judge shall take the throne,*
> *And when the cause is fully pleaded,*
> *O Jesu Son of Mary, shield Thou my soul,*
> *O Michael fair, acknowledge my departure.*
> *O Jesu Son of Mary, shield Thou my soul.*

Today I will reflect upon doing my best in life.

September 26th

On this day in 1181 Saint Francis of Assisi was born. The son of a prosperous silk merchant, Francis lived an idle life of pleasure until undergoing a spiritual experience in his early 20s. This led him to renounce all worldly things and dedicate his life to helping the poor.

He founded the Franciscan Order of Friars for men and the Poor Clares for women. He also founded the Third Order of St Francis for those unable to follow the itinerant preacher's life. Famous for his gentleness and love of animals, Francis is one of Christianity's best loved saints.

The following prayer, part of the *Canticle of the Creatures*, was written towards the end of his life:

Praised be you, my Lord, with all your creatures,
especially Sir Brother Sun,
who is the day and through whom you give us light. And he is beauti-
    ful and radiant with great splendour;
and bears a likeness of you, Most High One.
Praised be you, my Lord, through Sister Moon and the stars:
in heaven you formed them clear and precious and beautiful.
Praised be you, my Lord, through Brother Wind;
and through the air, cloudy and serene, and every kind of weather,
through which you give sustenance to your creatures.

Today I ask that I may be as humble and loving as St Francis was.

September 27th

On this day in 1912 *Memphis Blues* by WC Handy was the first blues song to be published, from which sprang the jazz age and ultimately, the whole popular music phenomenon.

Known as the 'Father of the Blues', Handy grew up in the Deep South but later moved to New York. He became blind following an accidental fall from a subway platform in 1943. A much loved figure, more than eight hundred people attended his 84th birthday party at the Waldorf-Astoria Hotel. When he died in 1958, over 25,000 people went to his funeral in Harlem's Abyssinian Baptist Church and over 150,000 people gathered in the streets near the church to pay their respects.

Elvis Presley has great respect for the blues and three years before the death of WC Handy, Presley began making records in Memphis, Tennessee. *Heartbreak Hotel* became number one in the charts in 1956.

Here is the start of one of Handy's greatest songs that really gives a blues flavour – *Beale Street Blues*:

> *You'll see pretty browns in beautiful gowns*
> *You'll see tailor-mades and hand-me-downs*
> *You'll meet honest men and pick-pockets skilled*
> *You'll find that business never closes*
> *Till somebody gets killed*
> *If Beale Street could talk, if Beale Street could talk*
> *Married men would have to take their beds and walk*
> *Except one or two, who never drink booze*
> *And the blind man on the corner*
> *Who sings the Beale Street Blues.*

Today I give thanks for the joy that music brings to the world.

September 28th

On this day in 1934 the French film star and animal rights campaigner Brigitte Bardot was born. World famous as a sex symbol in the 50s and 60s, she made nearly 50 films, many in the French language. Bardot became a 'national treasure' in France and modelled for the face of Marianne, the emblem of the French Republic and the goddess of reason and liberty.

In later life, Bardot retired to her villa at St Tropez where she continues to campaign for animal rights, particularly endangered species, saying: "I gave my beauty and my youth to men. I am going to give my wisdom and experience to animals." She has also got herself into trouble by speaking out against immigration and has been fined several times for criticising certain Muslim practices.

Here is a poem about a beautiful woman, Sylvia. Shakespeare wrote it four hundred years before Bardot was born, but it could have been written for her:

> *Who is Silvia? What is she?*
> *That all our swains commend her?*
> *Holy, fair, and wise is she;*
> *The heaven such grace did lend her,*
> *That she might admirèd be.*
> *Is she kind as she is fair?*
> *For beauty lives with kindness.*
> *Love doth to her eyes repair,*
> *To help him of his blindness,*
> *And, being helped, inhabits there.*
> *Then to Silvia let us sing,*
> *That Silvia is excelling;*
> *She excels each mortal thing*
> *Upon the dull earth dwelling:*
> *To her let us garlands bring.*

Today I give thanks for beauty of all kinds.

September 29th

On this day in 1973 the English poet WH Auden died. A prolific writer and traveller who became for a while an American citizen and resident, he wrote around four hundred poems mainly on the themes of love or politics.

Auden moved in the artistic circles of the time which included Stephen Spender, Cecil Day-Lewis, Christopher Isherwood, Benjamin Britten and TS Eliot. His private life included affairs with a number of men and though he seemed to yearn for a lifetime relationship, it never happened. He embraced spirituality particularly through the works of Kierkegaard and Niebuhr.

From 1956 to 1961 he was Professor of Poetry at Oxford University. His writing is notable for its direct expression of feelings and appeals to a wide audience. His poem *Funeral Blues* had a huge impact in the film Four Weddings and a Funeral.

The poet AE Housman was a big influence on Auden and he would have known poems such as this one, *Because I Liked You*:

Because I liked you better
    Than suits a man to say,
It irked you, and I promised
    To throw the thought away.

To put the world between us
    We parted, stiff and dry;
'Good-bye,' said you, ' forget me.'
    'I will, no fear', said I.

If here, where clover whitens
    The dead man's knoll, you pass,
And no tall flower to meet you
    Starts in the trefoiled grass,

Halt by the headstone naming
    The heart no longer stirred,
And say the lad that loved you
    Was one that kept his word.

Today I pray that I will be able to express my feelings when I need to.

September 30th

On this day in 1399 King Richard II of England was forced to abdicate in favour of his cousin, Henry Bolingbroke. Acceding to the throne at the age of ten, Richard had played a major part in suppressing the Peasants Revolt, when aged only 14.

Henry Bolingbroke later successfully challenged King Richard's right to the throne, deposed him and locked him up in Pontefract Castle where he died in February 1400; he is believed to have been starved to death. Much of our view of Richard comes from Shakespeare's play and most historians agree that it gives a fairly accurate account of the events.

Here is part of old, dying John of Gaunt's speech – lines that can make strong men weep:

> This royal throne of kings, this scepter'd isle,
> This earth of majesty, this seat of Mars,
> This other Eden, demi-paradise,
> This fortress built by Nature for herself
> Against infection and the hand of war,
> This happy breed of men, this little world,
> This precious stone set in the silver sea,
> Which serves it in the office of a wall,
> Or as a moat defensive to a house,
> Against the envy of less happier lands,
> This blessed plot, this earth, this realm, this England.
> This land of such dear souls, this dear, dear land,
> Dear for her reputation through the world,
> Is now leased out – I die pronouncing it,
> Like to a tenement or pelting-farm.
> That England that was wont to conquer others
> Hath made a shameful conquest of itself.

Today I give thanks for the love I have for my country.

October 1st

On this day in 1867 Karl Marx published his book *Das Kapital*. He saw capitalism as the exploitation of labour by those holding the productive capital assets – the employers. Given his trenchant views on capitalism, some people have been surprised to learn that Karl Marx himself was not above playing the stock market.

In 1864, according to historical documents, share deals in London netted the 'Father of Communism' the equivalent of £15,000. The money for his venture into capitalism was borrowed from his factory-owning comrade, Friedrich Engels.

Marx is quoted as telling friends, with breathtaking political incorrectness: 'It doesn't take much time to do this, and, if you are willing to risk a little bit, you can grasp money away from your opponents.'

Marx wrote several sonnets to his wife, Jenny Von Westphalen, including this, *Concluding Sonnet to Jenny*:

> One more thing to you, Child, I must tell:
> Gay this farewell poem, my singing's end;
> These last waves of silver throb and swell
> That my Jenny's breath its music lend.
> Swift as over gulf and looming fell,
> Through cascade and forest land,
> Life's fleet hours shall hasten on until
> Pure perfection's end in you they find.
> Bravely clad in flowing robes of fire,
>   Proud uplifted heart transformed by light,
> Master now, from bonds released entire,
> Firmly do I tread through spaces free,
> Shatter pain before your visage bright,
> While the dreams flash out towards Life's Tree.

Today I ask that people of all political hues may coexist happily.

October 2nd

On this day in 1968 the great French painter, sculptor and conceptual artist Marcel Duchamp died. He will always be remembered for his 'fountain' which is in fact a urinal, what he called a 'readymade'.

Duchamp wanted to move away from purely visual art into the idea behind it. He liked pop art: as he said in 1964, "If you take a Campbell soup can and repeat it 50 times, you are not interested in the retinal image. What interests you is the concept that wants to put 50 Campbell soup cans on a canvas."

After 1923, Duchamp's main interest was chess which he played obsessively, seeing it as a pure form of art which he sometimes used in other art works. In 1968, he played an artistically important chess match with the composer John Cage, at a concert entitled "Reunion". Music was produced by a series of photoelectric cells underneath the chessboard, triggered sporadically by normal game play. The French avant-garde poet René Daumal knew Duchamp.

Here is one of his poems, Poem from *Mount Analogue*:

> One cannot stay on the summit forever –
> One has to come down again.
> So why bother in the first place? Just this.
> What is above knows what is below –
> But what is below does not know what is above.
> One climbs, one sees –
> One descends and sees no longer
> But one has seen!
> There is an art of conducting one's self in
> The lower regions by the memory of
> What one saw higher up.
> When one can no longer see,
> One does at least still know.

Today I ask that I will be able to appreciate art with an open mind.

October 3rd

On this day in 1886 Alain-Fournier was born, author of the strange and wonderful novel *Le Grand Meaulnes*. The book has had a cult following – Scott Fitzgerald admired it so much he imitated its title and some of the story in *The Great Gatsby*; Jack Kerouac in *On the Road* has his hero Sal Paradise carry the book in his travels across America. The bittersweet story of adolescent friendship, betrayal and disappointment is drawn partly from the author's own life experience.

Alain-Fournier was killed aged 33 at the start of the First World War

In his novel, the hero Augustin Meaulnes meets by chance a beautiful young woman called Yvonne de Galais whom he searches for and longs to find again, This mirrors the real life experience of Alain-Fournier himself.

The plot is intricate and the mood one of sadness and yearning for lost dreams and friendships. John Fowles claimed it informed everything he wrote. "I know it has many faults," he said, "yet it has haunted me all my life."

Here is a taste:

> *"I don't even know who you are" she said at last. She spoke each word in an even tone, with the same emphasis on every one, but saying the last in a softer voice . . . then her face became impassive again; she bit her lip a little and her blue eyes stared into the distance. "And I don't know your name either" Meaulnes replied.*
> *They were following a path in the open and, some distance away, could see the guests gathering around a house isolated in the open countryside. "That's Franz's house" the young woman said, "I have to leave you . . ." She paused, looking at him for a moment with a smile, and said: "My name? I'm Mademoiselle Yvonne de Galais." Then she was gone.*

Today I ask that I will always be grateful for friendship.

October 4th

On this day in 1880 the American writer and journalist Damon Runyon was born. Famous for his portrayal of the Manhattan underworld and its colourful characters in the prohibition era, the guys and dolls that featured in nearly all his stories were drawn from real life observations, written at a time when dialogue and character were all important and plot often an irrelevance.

Here is an example of the Runyon effect – the perpetual present tense, the absence of conditional moods, the stilted, over-elaborate attempt at precision; all told by the nameless and anxious Narrator, with his warily formal diction and his cautious good manners: "This Rusty Charley is what is known as a gorill, because he is known often to carry a gun in his pants pocket and sometimes to shoot people down as dead as door nails with it, if he does not like the way they wear their hats – and Rusty Charley is very critical about hats".

Runyon captured a time of violence, bootlegging and gambling in the US and turned it into comedy. His prose, once seen, is unforgettable: "The race is not always to the swift, nor the battle to the strong, but that's how the smart money bets."

A fan of horse racing, he might have known Banjo Paterson's famous poem, *Pardon the Son of Reprieve*, that ends:

> And if they have racing hereafter,
> (And who is to say they will not?)
> When the cheers and the shouting and laughter
> Proclaim that the battle grows hot;
> As they come down the racecourse a-steering,
> He'll rush to the front, I believe;
> And you'll hear the great multitude cheering
> For Pardon, the son of Reprieve.

Today I pray that I may find comedy even in the darkest situations.

October 5th

O n this day in 1582, October 5th 'Never Happened'. Under the urging of the Catholic Church, much of Europe replaced the Julian calendar with the Gregorian calendar; the switch required the ten days after October 4th to be skipped. People panicked, thinking the government was robbing them of a part of their lives.

The Gregorian calendar at that time was running ten days ahead of the Julian because of the different ways that leap years had been calculated over the centuries. So on the Gregorian basis October 4th became October 14th. People at the time found this hard to understand. One can certainly sympathise – it is not easy to separate the concepts. Folk were a little more simple back then and could not separate the concepts of measuring time (the calendar) and time itself (you'll die when you die, regardless of what church and state decide to call that day).

Today's poem is entitled *It Never Happened* (Anon):

It never happened,
That I loved this much,
It never happened,
Because, in the past, I didn't love,
But I played the role of love,
It never happened,
I didn't know any woman before you,
That defeated me, took my weapons,
That beat me, in my own kingdom,
That took the masks off of my face,
It never happened, my lady,
That I tasted fire, and burning.

Be sure, my lady,
Thousands will love you,
And you will receive love letters,
But you will never find, after me,
A man that loves with the honesty,
You will never find it,
Not in the west, Nor in the east.

Today I ask that I will make the best possible use of the time that I have and live each day as if it is my last.

October 6th

On this day in 1887 the famous Swiss architect Le Corbusier was born (his real name was Charles-Édouard Jeanneret-Gris. Originally interested in painting as well as architecture, Le Corbusier first embraced Cubism before evolving his own style, which he called Purism.

He became particularly interested in urban living and large scale constructions such as tower blocks, the most famous of which being the 'Unité d'habitation' in Marseille, designed in the 1950s. He later took to designing cities for several million inhabitants, some very futuristic indeed. They did not meet with universal approval. He was however much in demand and his death in 1967 was notable for the tributes that came from all parts of the world.

This poem is about London and its buildings. It is by Scottish poet William McGonagall, often dubbed 'the worst Poet of the English language' for his (supposedly) unintentional mangling of metre, mood and vocabulary. See what you think:

> As I stood upon London Bridge and viewed the mighty throng
> Of thousands of people in cabs and busses rapidly whirling along,
> All furiously driving to and fro,
> Up one street and down another as quick as they could go:
> Then I was struck with the discordant sound of human voices there,
> Which seemed to me like wild geese cackling in the air:
> And the river Thames is a most beautiful sight,
> To see the steamers sailing upon it by day and by night.
> And the Tower of London is most gloomy to behold,
> And the crown of England lies there, begemmed with precious stones
>   and gold;
> King Henry the Sixth was murdered there by the Duke of Glo'ster,
> And when he killed him with his sword he called him an impostor

Today I give thanks for variety in everything and the freedom of choice that should be the right of all.

October 7th

On this day in 1885 the Danish physicist and peace campaigner Niels Bohr was born. In 1922 he won the Nobel Prize for his work on atom structures. Bohr was a friend of Einstein and was well known for his quirky sense of humour and witty sayings such as: "Prediction is always very difficult, especially about the future."

When a friend saw a horseshoe over the door of Bohr's country cabin, he said in mock astonishment, "Surely you don't believe in that old superstition". "No," said Bohr, "but they say it works even if you don't believe in it."

Like most great scientists, Bohr was a deep thinker, saying for example: "Every great and deep difficulty bears in itself its own solution. It forces us to change our thinking in order to find it."

Today's poem is by the avant-garde French poet René Daumal. I think that the world peace campaigner Niels Bohr would have appreciated it, *La Peau de la Lumiére*:

Light skin clothing this world is without
Thickness and I can see the deep night of all
The same body in varied clothes and the light of myself.
It was this night that even the mask of sunshine cannot hide.
I am the watcher of the night, the listener of silence
Because silence also wears a sounding skin
And each way has its night. Like myself I am my night.
I'm the thinker of non-being and splendour
I am the father of death.
She is the mother that I call up from the perfect
Mirror of the night
I'm the man upside down
My word is a hole in the silence. I know
Disillusionment I destroy what I become
I kill what I love.

Today I pray for all the people in the world and especially the original thinkers – perhaps they will find something to help us all.

October 8th

On this day in 1970 the Russian dissident author Alexander Solzhenitsyn was awarded the Nobel Prize for Literature. Among his best known books are *One Day in the Life of Ivan Denisovich* and *The Gulag Archipelago* which drew upon his experiences in forced labour camps.

Although a loyal Red Army officer during the Second World War, he was accused of anti-Soviet propaganda in 1945 and sentenced to eight years in a labour camp. Following the demise of Stalin, Solzhenitsyn was freed by Khrushchev and was even allowed in 1962, to publish *One Day in the Life of Ivan Denisovich* within the Soviet Union, where it became a huge best seller despite its politically charged themes. This publication was truly remarkable; fellow Russian Boris Pasternak's novel Doctor Zhivago had to be smuggled out of the Soviet Union to an Italian publisher, only five years earlier.

Although exiled from the Soviet Union in 1974, he was allowed back twenty years later and died in Moscow in 2008, aged 89. Much of his life had been characterised by exile.

This poem, by American poet Harold Hart-Crane, gives some of that feel, *Exile*:

> My hands have not touched pleasure since your hands,
> No, nor my lips freed laughter since ' farewell'
> And with the day, distance again expands
> Voiceless between us, as an uncoiled shell.
>
> Yet, love endures, though starving and alone.
> A dove's wings clung about my heart each night
> With surging gentleness, and the blue stone
> Set in the tryst-ring has but worn more bright.

Today I ask to feel sympathy with all exiles and to offer them the hand of welcome.

October 9th

On this day in 1967 Ernesto "Che" Guevara, Marxist revolutionary and physician, was executed in Bolivia, aged 39. Guevara was an Argentinian with part Irish ancestry. His father said "the thing to note is that in my son's veins flowed the blood of the Irish rebels".

Born into a middle class family in Buenos Aires, Guevara studied medicine and was a keen rugby player and golfer. He travelled widely in South America and was radicalised by seeing so much poverty and disease. In his 20s he travelled to Cuba to join Castro's revolution.

He was instrumental in getting the Russians to site their missiles in Cuba, which resulted in the missile crisis of 1964. Guevara left Cuba in 1965 to foment revolution abroad, and was captured in Bolivia by CIA-assisted forces and summarily executed.

Today's poem is by Lord Byron, another traveller and revolutionary sympathiser, *The Destruction of Sennecharib*:

> *The Assyrian came down like the wolf on the fold,*
> *And his cohorts were gleaming in purple and gold;*
> *And the sheen of their spears was like stars on the sea,*
> *When the blue wave rolls nightly on deep Galilee.*
> *Like the leaves of the forest when Summer is green,*
> *That host with their banners at sunset were seen:*
> *Like the leaves of the forest when Autumn hath blown,*
> *That host on the morrow lay withered and strown.*
> *For the Angel of Death spread his wings on the blast,*
> *And breathed in the face of the foe as he passed;*
> *And the widows of Ashur are loud in their wail,*
> *And the idols are broke in the temple of Baal;*
> *And the might of the Gentile, unsmote by the sword,*
> *Hath melted like snow in the glance of the Lord!*

Today I ask that there will always be people prepared to fight and die for the causes that they believe in.

October 10th

On this day in 1967 Brendan Behan's play *Borstal Boy*, based on his own life, was premiered in Dublin. The story depicts a young, fervently Republican Behan, imprisoned for his terrorist activities, who learns that he has a lot in common with his Protestant, British fellow prisoners.

Behan was also a poet, short story writer and novelist whose work was hugely successful. He learnt the Irish language while in prison and also lived in Paris. He was given to sayings such as: "I didn't turn to drink, drink turned on me", and "I have joined alcoholics anonymous – I am drinking under an assumed name!" Behan was a soldier in an armed struggle.

Today's soldier poem, written in 1863 by Irish-American bandleader Patrick Gilmore, is about the American Civil War:

> When Johnny comes marching home again
> Hurrah! Hurrah!
> We'll give him a hearty welcome then
> Hurrah! Hurrah!
> The men will cheer and the boys will shout
> The ladies they will all turn out
> And we'll all feel gay
> When Johnny comes marching home.
> The old church bell will peal with joy
> Hurrah! Hurrah!
> To welcome home our darling boy,
> Hurrah! Hurrah!
> Get ready for the Jubilee,
> Hurrah! Hurrah!
> And we'll all feel gay
> When Johnny comes marching home.

Today I will remember all those in prison that they may come to a better life.

October 11th

O n this day in 1963 the great French singer Édith Piaf died aged 47. Born Édith Giovanna Gassion in Belleville, Paris, her mother was an Italian café singer and her father was a street acrobat. Édith's parents soon abandoned her, and she was brought up by her grandmother, who ran a brothel.

She began to earn a precarious living as a street singer and in 1935 was discovered by Louis Leplée, a successful club owner and soon after she was famous. Her nervous energy and small stature inspired the nickname La Môme Piaf (The little Sparrow).

Here is a poem by Khalil Gibran about children and how to treat them:

And a woman who held a babe against her bosom said, 'Speak to us of Children.'
And he said:
Your children are not your children.
They are the sons and daughters of Life's longing for itself.
They come through you but not from you,
And though they are with you, yet they belong not to you.
You may give them your love but not your thoughts.
For they have their own thoughts.
You may house their bodies but not their souls,
For their souls dwell in the house of tomorrow, which you cannot visit, not even in your dreams.
You may strive to be like them, but seek not to make them like you.
For life goes not backward nor tarries with yesterday.
You are the bows from which your children as living arrows are sent forth.

Today I will remember the disadvantaged and the destitute, that their lot may be improved.

October 12th

On this day in 1492 Christopher Columbus made his first landfall in the new world on the island he named San Salvador. In spite of making the rather large mistake of thinking he had arrived in China, a view that he never changed, Columbus became one of history's most famous names.

Born in Genoa, he was clever enough as a young man to see the possibility of a western approach to the East Indies because, unlike many at the time, he accepted that the earth was round, rather than flat.

Here is part of a poem by John Donne, written about one hundred years after Columbus' first voyage, which uses the event as a metaphor for discovery of a different kind – in love-making, *On his mistress going to bed*:

> Licence my roving hands, and let them go,
> Before, behind, between, above, below.
> O my America! My new-found-land,
> My kingdom, safeliest when with one man mann'd,
> My Mine of precious stones, My Empirie,
> How blest am I in this discovering thee!
> To enter in these bonds, is to be free;
> Then where my hand is set, my seal shall be.
>
> Like pictures, or like books' gay coverings made
> For lay-men, are all women thus array'd.
> Themselves are mystic books, which only we
> (Whom their imputed grace will dignify)
> Must see reveal'd. Then since that I may know;
> As liberally, as to a Midwife, shew
> Thy self: cast all, yea, this white linen hence,
> There is no penance due to innocence.
>   To teach thee, I am naked first; why then
> What needst thou have more covering than a man.

Today I pray that the joys of discovery can be put to good use.

October 13th

On this day in AD 54 the Roman Emperor Tiberius Claudius Caesar Augustus Germanicus died, supposedly poisoned. Known today as Claudius, he was the fourth Roman emperor and one of the best.

Born into the imperial family and partly disabled by a deformed leg, he was not seen as a threat when his predecessor Caligula was murdered. Found hiding after the event by the Praetorian Guard, he was proclaimed emperor on the spot.

The story was told by the English poet Robert Graves in his 1934 novel *I Claudius*. His rule turned out to be wise and effective and Rome was a much more powerful nation when he died. It was 25 years after his death that Mount Vesuvius erupted, burying the towns of Pompeii and Herculaneum.

Here is part of a poem about Pompeii by Thomas Babington Macaulay, *Pompeii*:

> Well have they mouldering walls, Pompeii, known,
> Decked in those charms, and by that rage o'erthrown.
> Sad City, gayly dawned thy latest day,
> And poured its radiance on the scene as gay.
> The leaves scarce rustled in the sighing breeze;
> In azure dimples curled the sparkling seas,
> And as the golden tide of light they quaffed,
> Campania's sunny meads and vineyards laughed,
> While gleamed each lichened oak and giant pine
> On the far sides of swarthy Apennine.
> Then mirth and music through Pompeii rung;
> Then verdant wreaths on all her portals hung;
> Her sons with solemn rite and jocund lay,
> Hailed the glad splendours of that festal day

Today I ask that I shall strive to do my best, whatever my disabilities.

October 14th

On this day in 1924, *Winnie the Pooh* by AA Milne was published. Milne wrote the stories about Pooh, Piglet and the rest for his young son, Christopher Robin Milne.

To enter their little world is to feel happy and secure: "When you wake up in the morning, Pooh," said Piglet at last, "what's the first thing you say to yourself?" "What's for breakfast?" said Pooh. "What do you say, Piglet?" "I say, I wonder what's going to happen exciting today" said Piglet. Pooh nodded thoughtfully. "It's the same thing, he said."

After the huge success of the books, Milne became increasingly frustrated, wanting recognition as a more serious writer. This never happened and he will always be remembered as the creator of the magical world of Christopher Robin.

Today's poem is about childhood – *The Swing*, by Robert Louis Stevenson:

> How do you like to go up in a swing,
> Up in the air so blue?
> Oh, I do think it the pleasantest thing
> Ever a child can do!
>
> Up in the air and over the wall,
> Till I can see so wide,
> River and trees and cattle and all
> Over the countryside –
>
> Till I look down on the garden green,
> Down on the roof so brown –
> Up in the air I go flying again,
> Up in the air and down!

Today I ask that I will be grateful for the small and simple things in life.

October 15th

On this day in 1844 the great German philosopher Friedrich Nietzsche was born. A strong atheist, he is chiefly remembered for his savage indictments of religion: "Certainly the Christian religion is an antiquity projected into our times from remote prehistory; and the fact that the claim is believed – whereas one is otherwise so strict in examining pretensions – is perhaps the most ancient piece of this heritage."

Such views on religion contrast with his strongly held views on the integrity of humanity and man's capacity for shaping his own destiny. He is often called the Father of Existentialism: 'In every Now, being begins; round every Here rolls the sphere There. The centre is everywhere. Bent is the path of eternity.'

Today's poem is by way of relief from such heavyweight thinking, *Love's Philosophy* by Percy Bysshe Shelley:

> *Fountains mingle with the river*
> *And the rivers with the ocean,*
> *The winds of heaven mix for ever*
> *With a sweet emotion;*
> *Nothing in the world is single;*
> *All things by a law divine*
> *In one spirit meet and mingle.*
> *Why not I with thine? –*
> *See the mountains kiss high heaven*
> *And the waves clasp one another;*
> *No sister-flower would be forgiven*
> *If it disdained its brother;*
> *And the sunlight clasps the earth*
> *And the moonbeams kiss the sea:*
> *What is all this sweet work worth*
> *If thou kiss not me?*

Today I ask that I will keep it simple and not complicate my world views unnecessarily.

October 16th

On this day in 1854 the Irish poet and playwright Oscar Wilde was born. London's most popular dramatist of his day and lionised by society, he is also remembered for the sudden fall from grace that happened in 1895 when he lost his libel case against the Marquis of Queensberry, father of Wilde's lover, Lord Alfred Douglas, who had called him a 'sodomite'.

Wilde was himself then prosecuted by the crown for gross indecency and served a prison sentence, from which he emerged a broken man to spend his last years in France, never returning to England or Ireland.

He died almost destitute in Paris in 1900, his last words: "Either that wallpaper goes or I do".

Here is one of his poems, *Chanson*:

> *A ring of gold and a milk-white dove*
> *Are goodly gifts for thee,*
> *And a hempen rope for your own love*
> *To hang upon a tree.*
> *For you a House of Ivory*
> *(Roses are white in the rose-bower)!*
> *A narrow bed for me to lie*
> *(White, O white, is the hemlock flower)!*
> *Myrtle and jessamine for you*
> *(O the red rose is fair to see)!*
> *For me the cypress and the rue*
> *(Fairest of all is rose-mary)!*
> *For you three lovers of your hand*
> *(Green grass where a man lies dead)!*
> *For me three paces on the sand*
> *(Plant lilies at my head)!*

Today I ask that I may always look for the good in people and be grateful for the joy that they try to bring to the world.

October 17th

On this day in 1651 the prince and future King Charles II fled England following the defeat of his forces at the Battle of Worcester. The story of the young heir to the throne who hid in the oak tree at Boscobel while enemy forces hunted for him, and his subsequent wanderings for the next six weeks, dressed as a servant, before escaping to France in a coal boat.

Charles never forgot those who helped him escape. Less romantic was the fate of several of those who had signed the death warrant for his father's execution in 1649. He hunted them down remorselessly and, on this very day in 1660, nine regicides were hung, drawn and quartered in London

Charles was always popular with the ladies and here is part of a poem by Andrew Marvell about love making, *To his Coy Mistress*:

> *Had we but world enough, and time,*
> *This coyness, Lady, were no crime*
> *We would sit down and think which way*
> *To walk and pass our long love's day.*
>
> *But at my back I always hear*
> *Time's wingèd chariot hurrying near;*
> *And yonder all before us lie*
> *Deserts of vast eternity.*
> *Thy beauty shall no more be found,*
> *Nor, in thy marble vault, shall sound*
> *My echoing song: then worms shall try*
> *That long preserved virginity,*
> *And your quaint honour turn to dust,*
> *And into ashes all my lust:*
> *The grave 's a fine and private place,*
> *But none, I think, do there embrace.*

Today I ask that I will always show gratitude to those that helped me but not show revenge to those that harmed me.

October 18th

On this day in 1922 the British Broadcasting Corporation was founded. Originally a consortium of private companies, some of whom were manufacturers of wireless sets, the BBC was granted the first public broadcasting licence in Britain.

Head of the corporation was a Scottish Calvinist, John Reith, later Lord Reith. After a rocky start, the BBC was given a boost by the general strike of 1926, when newspapers could not be published. In 1927 the BBC was given status by a royal charter and has been a major force in the land ever since.

Today the corporation broadcasts around the world, on both radio and TV, and employs over 23,000 people. By the 1930s and 40s, the BBC was an integral part of most middle class lives. It played a vital part during the Second World War in uniting and informing the country.

Here is a poem by Rabindranath Tagore, *Baby's World*, about a young view of the world:

I wish I could take a quiet corner in the heart of my baby's very Own world.
I know it has stars that talk to him, and a sky that stoops
Down to his face to amuse him with its silly clouds and rainbows.
Those who make believe to be dumb, and look as if they never
Could move, come creeping to his window with their stories and with
Trays crowded with bright toys.
I wish I could travel by the road that crosses baby's mind,
And out beyond all bounds;
Where messengers run errands for no cause between the kingdoms
Of kings of no history;
Where Reason makes kites of her laws and flies them, the Truth
Sets Fact free from its fetters.

Today I ask that I will be a useful and caring member of society.

October 19th

On this day in 1781, the British Army under General Charles Cornwallis surrendered at Yorktown, Virginia, thus ending the Revolutionary War. Despite the images of several famous paintings of the event, Cornwallis was not present at the surrender, claiming to be ill.

The war was a disaster for England, though the loss of the American colonies was soon made up for by conquests in India and the annexation of the recently discovered Australasia.

France, the colonists' ally, played a major part in the defeat of the English – some French leaders, such as the Marquis de Lafayette, went on to play major roles in the French Revolution some ten years later. Cornwallis was undaunted by the setback at Yorktown and went on to receive a knighthood and become Governor General of India.

Here is part of the poem *Yorktown*, by American poet John Greenleaf Whittier, writing roughly one hundred years after the event. Not one of his best perhaps, but he was making a point:

> *From Yorktown's ruins, ranked and still,*
> *Two lines stretch far o'er vale and hill:*
> *Who curbs his steed at head of one?*
> *Hark! The low murmur: Washington!*
> *Who bends his keen, approving glance,*
> *Where down the gorgeous line of France*
> *Shine knightly star and plume of snow?*
> *Thou too art victor, Rochambeau!*
> *The earth which bears this calm array*
> *Shook with the war-charge yesterday,*
> *Ploughed deep with hurrying hoof and wheel,*
> *Shot-sown and bladed thick with steel . . .*

Today I areflect on the example of Yorktown as a help to those seeking freedom.

October 20th

On this day in 1854 the French poet Arthur Rimbaud was born. Rimbaud was born a country boy in the Ardennes in Northern France. He went to Paris as a teenager and was befriended by the older, married and decadent poet Paul Verlaine. The two fell in love and ran away together, causing great scandal. Both were heavy alcohol and drug users and the relationship soon went sour. It finally ceased when Verlaine fired a revolver at Rimbaud, slightly wounding him – for this he was later imprisoned.

Rimbaud felt that his inspiration came from excess and degradation, as he tried to explain in a letter: 'I'm now making myself as scummy as I can. Why? I want to be a poet, and I'm working at turning myself into a seer. You won't understand any of this, and I'm almost incapable of explaining it to you. The idea is to reach the unknown by the derangement of all the senses. It involves enormous suffering, but one must be strong and be a born poet. It's really not my fault.'

Many poets have sought inspiration this way; Dylan Thomas called himself 'the Rimbaud of Cwmdonkin Drive'. Although he lived to the age of 37, he wrote all his poetry before he was 21. The brief firework that was his genius – its flowering and sudden extinction, still astonishes us. Here is an example, *Flowers*:

> From a terrace of gold – among threads of silk, grey gauze, green
> velvets and crystal discs that darken like bronze in the sun – I
> watch the foxglove open on a carpet of silver filigree, eyes and hair.
> Yellow gold coins sprinkled on agate, mahogany columns supporting
> an emerald dome, bunches of white satin and fine sprays of rubies
> surround the rose of water.
> Like a god with vast blue eyes and snowy forms, sea and sky draw
> hosts of young and vigorous roses to the terraces of marble.

Today I give thanks for the appearance of genius in our mundane lives.

October 21st

On this day in 1772 the poet Samuel Taylor Coleridge was born. A huge influence on later poets, he was a friend of Wordsworth, becoming a leading figure in the Romantic Movement.

Coleridge was a notorious opium addict and his famous poems, *Kubla Khan* and the *Rime of the Ancient Mariner*, were largely written while under its influence. The extraordinary imagery of his opium-laden imagination is inimitable and has enhanced the English language. Sadly, in his later life, opium became a huge albatross round the poet's neck and he spent the last 18 years of his life living in the home of a London doctor who helped him battle his addiction.

Here is a beautiful Coleridge poem, composed in an earlier and probably happier, time of life – *Reflections on Having Left a Place of Retirement*:

> In the open air
> Our Myrtles blossom'd; and across the porch
> Thick Jasmins twined: the little landscape round
> Was green and woody, and refresh'd the eye.
> It was a spot which you might aptly call
> The Valley of Seclusion!
> I was constrain'd to quit you. Was it right,
> While my unnumber'd brethren toil'd and bled,
> That I should dream away the entrusted hours
> On rose-leaf beds, pampering the coward heart
> With feelings all too delicate for use?
> I therefore go, and join head, heart, and hand,
> Active and firm, to fight the bloodless fight
> Of Science, Freedom, and the Truth in Christ.
> Yet oft when after honourable toil
> Rests the tir'd mind, and waking loves to dream
> My Spirit shall revisit thee, dear Cot!

Today I ask that I shall be able to live my life free of all mood altering drugs.

October 22nd

On this day in 1964 the French philosopher and writer Jean Paul Sartre refused to accept the Nobel Prize for literature. Sartre refused the prize saying that he always declined official honours and that "a writer should not allow himself to be turned into an institution".

Sartre popularised Existentialism though the ideas originated from 19th century thinkers such as Nietzsche and Kierkegaard who proposed that each individual – not society or religion – is solely responsible for giving meaning to life and living it passionately and sincerely, "authentically".

As He put it: "Man can will nothing unless he has first understood that he must count on no one but himself; that he is alone, abandoned on earth in the midst of his infinite responsibilities, without help, with no other aim than the one he sets himself, with no other destiny than the one he forges for himself on this earth."

This poem by WB Yeats seems to say there is satisfaction in simply being old with memories, *When You Are Old*:

> When you are old and grey and full of sleep,
> And nodding by the fire, take down this book,
> And slowly read, and dream of the soft look
> Your eyes had once, and of their shadows deep;
> How many loved your moments of glad grace,
> And loved your beauty with love false or true,
> But one man loved the pilgrim soul in you,
> And loved the sorrows of your changing face;
> And bending down beside the glowing bars,
> Murmur, a little sadly, how Love fled
> And paced upon the mountains overhead
> And hid his face amid a crowd of stars.

Today I ask that I will be able to handle pessimism and negativity with understanding of myself.

October 23rd

On this day in 1958 the Russian author Boris Pasternak was awarded the Nobel Prize for literature for his novel *Doctor Zhivago*, that had to be smuggled out of the Soviet Union for publication. The CIA was instrumental in making this happen, because they saw the impact it would have at the height of the Cold War.

On 25 October, Pasternak sent a telegram to the Swedish Academy: "Infinitely grateful, touched, proud, surprised, overwhelmed." It was a huge embarrassment for the Soviets.

That same day, the Literary Institute in Moscow demanded that all its students sign a petition denouncing Pasternak and his novel. They were further ordered to join a "spontaneous" demonstration demanding Pasternak's exile from the Soviet Union. Immense pressure was put upon the author by the authorities and he eventually decided to withdraw his acceptance of the prize (though the Nobel committee never withdrew the award).

Pasternak was first of all a Russian and wanted to stay that way – there was never any question of voluntary exile. He was later tried and persecuted by the state but never imprisoned. He died in 1960 of lung cancer. Although chiefly famous for his *Doctor Zhivago*, Pasternak considered himself a poet.

Here is his beautiful description of the essence of poetry:

> It is a steeply rising whistle
> It is the cracking of squeezed icicles
> It is frozen leaves through the night
> It is two nightingales singing a duel
> It is the stifled sweet pea plant
> It is the tears of the world on a shoulder.

Today I give thanks for the bravery of those who are prepared to stand up against persecution and thus give inspiration to others.

October 24th

On this day in 1931 the American gangster Alphonse (Al) Capone was sentenced to 11 years in jail for tax evasion. Capone had been lauded as a sort of Robin Hood figure in Chicago for some time, however the public's view of him changed after the St Valentine's Day massacre in 1929.

Federal lawmen had been after him for years. In prison, Capone became increasingly psychotic and began to be haunted by the ghost of James Clark, a massacre victim. Other inmates reported that they could hear Capone screaming in his cell begging 'Jimmy' to go away and leave him alone. Capone died of syphilis in 1947.

Today, Chicago is no longer the bootleg capital of old. Thousands fly daily into its famous O'Hare airport, named after World War II hero, fighter pilot Lt Butch O'Hare, killed in action in 1942. Few travellers realise that Butch O'Hare was the son of 'Easy' Eddie O'Hare, Capone's notorious lawyer who, after years spent saving his client from the law by dubious means, finally turned informer and gave damning evidence that put Capone behind bars. Easy Eddie may have walked away with a lighter conscience but it all ended badly; in 1939, he was gunned down in the street in an act of revenge. In his pockets, besides a revolver and a rosary, was found this well-chosen poem, by Robert H Smith:

The clock of life is wound but once
And no man has the power
To tell just when the hands will stop,
At late or early hour;
Now is the only time you own,
Live, love, toil with a will;
Place no faith in time,
For the clock may soon be still.

Today I pray that I may be grateful for each day that comes, and live it as if it is my last.

October 25th

On this day in 1881 the painter Pablo Picasso was born in Malaga, Spain. The son of a Spanish art teacher, Picasso lived in Spain and France and also, for a short time, in London with Diaghilev's Russian Ballet in 1919, for whom he designed sets and costumes. During this time he stayed at the Savoy Hotel and even bought a Savile Row suit and bowler hat to 'be like an English gentleman'.

It was said that he changed his women as often as he changed painting styles. It is hard to disagree with his mistress Dora Maar's summation: "As an artist you are extraordinary but morally speaking, you are worthless". He was so multi-talented that one woman wrote to him "if I hear that you say Mass too, I shall not be surprised".

Opinions vary on his poetry. According to a story from Hemingway's first wife, Hadley, one evening when Picasso was at Gertrude Stein's flat, he read some of his poetry to the hushed group, none of whom dared say anything when he finished. There was a long silence. Finally Gertrude said, "Pablo, go home and paint." This poem is entitled *Art* by Herman Melville:

> In placid hours well-pleased we dream
> Of many a brave unbodied scheme.
> But form to lend, pulsed life create,
> What unlike things must meet and mate:
> A flame to melt – a wind to freeze;
> Sad patience – joyous energies;
> Humility – yet pride and scorn;
> Instinct and study; love and hate:
> Audacity – reverence. These must mate,
> And fuse with Jacob's mystic heart,
> To wrestle with the angel – Art.

Today I pray that I may appreciate modern art however much of a challenge this may be.

October 26th

On this day in 1950, Mother Theresa founded the Missionaries of Charity in India. Born in Albania, she left home at the age of 18 to join the Sisters of Loreto as a missionary. She never again saw her mother or sister.

Soon she was working in India with the Sisters and at the age of 40 she had a spiritual experience calling her to leave the convent and devote her life to living among the poor and the sick. The fourth vow of the Missionaries is to give 'wholehearted free service to the poorest of the poor.'

Mother Teresa was the recipient of numerous honours including the 1979 Nobel Peace Prize. In 2003, she was beatified as 'Blessed Teresa of Calcutta'. She preached and showed the promotion of unconditional love, never doubting her vocation.

This poem, by the Persian mystic poet Rumi, is about a time of vocation, *It is Your Turn Now*:

> *It is your turn now,*
> *you waited, you were patient.*
> *The time has come,*
> *for us to polish you.*
> *We will transform your inner pearl*
> *into a house of fire.*
> *You're a gold mine.*
> *Did you know that,*
> *hidden in the dirt of the earth?*
> *It is your turn now,*
> *to be placed in fire.*
> *Let us cremate your impurities.*

Today I am grateful to those who offer free service and unconditional love.

October 27th

On this day in 1932 The American poet and writer Sylvia Plath was born. Plath grew up in Boston and went to Cambridge University on a scholarship where she met and married British poet Ted Hughes. Their marriage was stormy and they separated after their two children Frieda and Nicholas were born.

Plath had a long history of depression and suicide attempts. She killed herself, while in London with her children. Plath had received acclaim for her writing after her first book of poetry, *The Colossus and Other Poems*, was published in 1960.

Her second book of poetry, *Ariel*, was published after her death and contains remarkable images of menace and mystery: "And I, Am the arrow, The dew that flies, Suicidal". The idea of death was recurrent in her poetry and in her only novel, *The Bell Jar*.

In 2003 a film called *Sylvia* was made about her tragic life, which received mixed reviews and an angry response from her family. There have been many poets who have flirted with the idea of madness and expressed it in their poetry.

Here is reclusive Emily Dickenson's poem, *Much Madness is Divinest Sense*:

> Much madness is divinest sense
> To a discerning eye.
> Much sense, the starkest madness –
> Tis the majority.t
> In this, as all, prevail –
> Assent, and you are sane.
> Demur, you're straightway dangerous
> And handled with a chain.

Today I pray for all those who, through desperation, are driven to end their lives.

October 28th

On this day in 1903 the English writer Evelyn Waugh was born. "The greatest novelist of my generation" is how Graham Greene, a great novelist himself, described him.

Some of the best-written and best-loved books of the 20th century came from his pen, such as *Brideshead Revisited, Decline and Fall, Scoop*, and *The Loved One*. Although his upbringing was fairly ordinary, through his Oxford education, Waugh developed a taste for the aristocracy and the life of country houses and London clubs.

Many of his books are fanciful embroiderings on his own experiences. He served with distinction throughout the Second World War, and a few years later suffered a mental breakdown. In later years his physical health deteriorated and he died at home of a heart attack aged 62, after morning mass. A good end for a staunch Catholic.

He felt strongly that a writer should take an active part in expressing opinions: "A writer must face the choice of becoming an artist or a prophet. He can shut himself up at his desk and selfishly seek pleasure in the perfecting of his own skill or he can pace about, dictating dooms and exhortations on the topics of the day."

Such directness puts me in mind of the old anonymous ditty:

> O, do not be discouraged, when
> You find your hopes brought down,
> And when you meet unwilling men
> Heed not their gloomy frown.
> Yield not to wild despair;
> Press on and give no quarter,
> In battle all is fair;
> We'll win, for we had orter.

Today I pray that I will be able to treat everyone with respect and if necessary, suffer fools gladly.

October 29th

On this day in 1618 the English adventurer and writer Sir Walter Raleigh was beheaded for allegedly plotting against King James I of England. Raleigh had risen rapidly in the favour of Queen Elizabeth I and was knighted in 1585. He was granted a royal patent to explore and colonise Virginia in North America. After Queen Elizabeth died in 1603, Raleigh was imprisoned in the Tower, for being involved in the so-called Main Plot (there were others) against King James I In 1616, he was released to lead a second expedition, to South America in search of gold. This was unsuccessful, and men under his command ransacked a Spanish outpost.

He returned to England and, to appease the Spanish, was arrested and executed in 1618. Raleigh is well known for promoting the smoking of tobacco in England. As King James had written one of the earliest known attacks on the smoking habit, it is perhaps not surprising that they did not get along. Raleigh was known for his charm and his poetry reflects this; here is Farewell to the Court:

> *Like truthless dreams, so are my joys expir'd,*
> *And past return are all my dandled days;*
> *My love misled, and fancy quite retir'd –*
> *Of all which pass'd the sorrow only stays.*
> *My lost delights, now clean from sight of land,*
> *Have left me all alone in unknown ways;*
> *My mind to woe, my life in fortune's hand –*
> *Of all which pass'd the sorrow only stays.*
> *As in a country strange, without companion,*
> *I only wail the wrong of death's delays,*
> *Whose sweet spring spent, whose summer well-nigh done*
> *Of all which pass'd only the sorrow stays.*
> *Whom care forewarns, ere age and winter cold,*
> *To haste me hence to find my fortune's fold.*

Today I will remember all those who are imprisoned for their political beliefs.

October 30th

On this day in 1938 the writer, director and actor Orson Welles panicked the USA with his radio broadcast of HG Wells' *War of the Worlds* about extraterrestrials landing on earth, which many people thought was real.

The publicity from the event made his name. He went on to make *Citizen Kane* in 1941, recognised as one of the greatest films ever made. Welles' career never progressed much after *Citizen Kane*.

The advent of television changed the entertainment industry – nobody wanted the egotistical, arrogant type of actor/director any more. Welles always said that he suffered from being told at a young age that he was perfect.

Today's poem by Gerard Manly Hopkins is about perfection, *The Habit of Perfection*:

> *Elected Silence, sing to me*
> *And beat upon my whorlèd ear,*
> *Pipe me to pastures still and be*
> *The music that I care to hear.*
>
> *Shape nothing, lips; be lovely-dumb:*
> *It is the shut, the curfew sent*
> *From there where all surrenders come*
> *Which only makes you eloquent.*
>
> *Be shellèd, eyes, with double dark*
> *And find the uncreated light:*
> *This ruck and reel which you remark*
> *Coils, keeps, and teases simple sight.*
>
> *And, Poverty, be thou the bride*
> *And now the marriage feast begun,*
> *And lily-coloured clothes provide*
> *Your spouse not laboured-at nor spun.*

Today I give thanks for the talents I possess and ask that I may never waste them.

October 31st

On this day in 1517 the German cleric Martin Luther published his *Ninety Five Theses* – he also nailed them to the door of All Saints church in Wittenberg. This started the Reformation, whereby the grip of the Catholic Church in Rome was broken in much of Europe, to be replaced by Protestantism. Luther was a Catholic priest and Professor of Theology at the University of Wittenberg. A Dominican friar named Johann Tetzel had been sent to Germany by the Pope to sell indulgences (pardon for sins) so as to raise money for the building of St Peter's church in Rome. Luther particularly objected to a saying attributed to Tetzel that: "As soon as the coin in the coffer rings, the soul into heaven springs".

The *Ninety Five Theses* were printed, and widely copied, making the protest one of the first in history to be aided by the printing press. Luther later married and had six children. He started the Reformation and changed the world.

He wrote many poems and hymns too, here is one:

> God is our refuge in distress,
> Our shield of hope through every care,
> Our Shepherd watching us to bless,
> And therefore will we not despair;
> Although the mountains shake,
> And hills their place forsake,
> And billows o'er them break
> Yet still will we not fear,
> For Thou, O God, art ever near.
> Then though the earth remove,
> And storms rage high above,
> And seas tempestuous prove,
> Yet still will we not fear,
> The Lord of Hosts is ever near.

Today I ask that I may be as steadfast in acting out my beliefs as Martin Luther was.

November 1st

On this day in 1512 Michelangelo Buonarroti completed painting the ceiling of the Sistine Chapel. Contrary to popular belief, he did not paint it lying on his back, but standing up. Michelangelo always considered himself above all to be a sculptor rather than a painter – he had never attempted a fresco before starting on the Sistine Chapel, which was a commission that he hated but completed at the behest of the Pope. Michelangelo lived simply, although he was by no means poor, and he looked after his family and those who worked for him well. His influence on Western art has been enormous. He had many male lovers in his life and wrote a lot of poetry on the subject of love. Here is a taste of his style, though in translation:

> *O night, O sweetest time, though black of hue,*
> *With peace you force all the restless work to end;*
> *Those who exalt you see and understand,*
> *And he is sound of mind who honours you.*
> *You cut the thread of tired thoughts, for so*
> *You offer calm in your moist shade; you send*
> *To this low sphere the dreams where we ascend*
> *Up to the highest, where I long to go.*
> *Shadow of death that brings to quiet close*
> *All miseries that plague the heart and soul,*
> *For those in pain the last and best of cures;*
> *You heal the flesh of its infirmities,*
> *Dry and our tears and shut away our toil,*
> *And free the good from wrath and fretting cares.*

Today I ask that I may do my best in whatever I turn my hand to.

November 2nd

On this day in 1755 Marie Antoinette was born, 15th child of the Holy Roman Emperor, Francis I, and future Queen of France. Married at the age of 14 to the Dauphin of France, the future King Louis XVI, her position appeared enviable. Though initially popular in France, she was soon perceived as a spendthrift, promiscuous and too sympathetic to France's enemies, especially Austria (her country of origin). Soon she was being called Madame Deficit (because of her spending), and worse, 'L'Autrichienne' (literally 'the Austrian woman') but also suggesting in its ending, the French word 'chienne' (bitch). Marie Antoinette syndrome is the condition where the sufferer's hair turns white as the result of a traumatic incident. This reportedly happened to her after the royal family's unsuccessful attempt to escape France, and their flight to Varennes, in 1791. Marie Antoinette was executed by guillotine on 16 October 1793. Her last words were "I am sorry sir, I did not mean to put it there" (she had trodden on the executioner's foot). Her extraordinary story of hubris and nemesis does not tell us what she was really like – we can only guess. I see her as a girl who made mistakes but one who loved her family, her friends and her children. Marie Antoinette was 38 when she was executed. For today's poem, I offer the last verse of *Ode on the Death of a Favourite Cat* by Thomas Gray which ends:

> *From hence, ye beauties, undeceiv'd*
> *Know, one false step is ne'er retriev'd,*
> *And be with caution bold.*
> *Not all that tempts your wandering eyes*
> *And heedless hearts, is lawful prize;*
> *Nor all, that glisters, gold.*

Today I ask that I will be able to translate my good intentions into deeds.

November 3rd

On this day in 1954 the French painter Henri Matisse died aged 84. He became part of the Fauvism movement and is especially noted for his use of colour. Later he became a friend of Picasso and the two men had a profound effect on the evolution of early twentieth century art. Both painted mostly women and still life. They were sometimes rivals but reminded friends, both living in the south of France in their later years. Matisse spent his last years doing collage, cutting out shapes with scissors that his assistants applied to the canvas under his close instruction. He found this easier than painting, due to the surgery that he had undergone. Matisse famously used poetry for inspiration and energy, saying that poetry is like oxygen,"just as when you leap out of bed you fill your lungs with fresh air". He used to read poems each morning before starting work in his studio, especially after his treatment for bowel cancer. Here is a poem that he might have read. It is by another Frenchman, Paul Valéry, who lived at the same time as Matisse, *La Feuille Blanche* (*The Blank Sheet*):

> In truth, a blank sheet
> Declares by the void
> That there is nothing as beautiful
> As that which does not exist.
> On the magic mirror of its white space,
> The soul sees before her the place of the miracles
> That we would bring to life with signs and lines.
> This presence of absence over-excites
> And at the same time paralyses the definitive act of the pen.
> There is in all beauty a forbiddance to touch,
> From which emanates I don't know what of sacred
> That stops the movement and puts the man
> On the point of acting in fear of himself.

Today I give thanks for the inspiration that poetry gives to many.

November 4th

On this day in 1922 the archaeologist Howard Carter discovered the tomb of Tutankhamen in Egypt. One of the most moving finds was a single cornflower placed in the king's hands, perhaps by his young widow. Egypt has provided a rich treasure trove of ancient Greek poetry that might otherwise have been lost. Some of sixth century BC Greek poetess Sappho's works for example, were found on fragments of papyrus that had been recycled into a kind of papier-mâché used to protect Egyptian mummies in their tombs. Here is one of Sappho's poems that could have been about Tutankhamen:

> *Blest as the immortal gods is he*
> *The youth whose eyes may look on thee*
> *Whose ears thy tongue's sweet melody*
> *May still devour.*
> *Thou smilest too – sweet smile whose charm*
> *Has struck my soul with wild alarm*
> *And when I see thee bids disarm*
> *Each vital power.*
> *Speechless I gaze: the flame within*
> *Runs swift o'er all my quivering skin:*
> *My eyeballs swim, with dizzy din*
> *My brain reels round.*
> *And cold drops fall; and tremblings frail*
> *Seize every limb and grassy pale*
> *I grow; and then, together fail*
> *Both sight and sound.*

Today I will reflect on the lasting power of love and not worry whether I will be remembered or not.

November 5th

On this day in 1605 the plot to blow up parliament and assassinate King James I of England, who was also King James VI of Scotland, was foiled. Guy Fawkes was found guarding the explosives. Asked what he was doing in possession of so much gunpowder, Fawkes answered: "to blow you Scotch beggars back to your native mountains." This brave comment earned the admiration of the King. Over the next few days, he was questioned and severely tortured, and eventually he confessed to the plot. Immediately before his execution, Fawkes jumped from the scaffold where he was to be hanged and broke his neck, thus avoiding the agony of the mutilation that would have followed. Each year the event is remembered with bonfires and fireworks where a 'Guy' in effigy is burnt. Fawkes was clearly a brave and daring man, if a rather foolish one. Today's poem by Rudyard Kipling is about being brave, *If*:

> If you can keep your head when all about you
> Are losing theirs and blaming it on you,
> If you can trust yourself when all men doubt you,
> But make allowance for their doubting too;
> If you can wait and not be tired by waiting,
> Or being lied about, don't deal in lies,
> Or being hated, don't give way to hating,
> And yet don't look too good, nor talk too wise
> If you can talk with crowds and keep your virtue,
> 'Or walk with Kings – nor lose the common touch,
> If neither foes nor loving friends can hurt you,
> If all men count with you, but none too much;
> If you can fill the unforgiving minute
> With sixty seconds' worth of distance run,
> Yours is the Earth and everything that's in it,
> And – which is more – you'll be a Man, my son!

Today I ask that I may be brave in what I set out to do.

On this day in 1860, Abraham Lincoln was elected 16th president of the United States. In the five extraordinary years that followed, he masterminded and won a Civil War and, in doing so, preserved the Union, abolished slavery, strengthened the Federal Government, and modernised the economy. He was assassinated in 1865 by the actor John Wilkes Booth, an angry and bitter Confederate, only days after calling for reconciliation between the two sides of the conflict. Lincoln was a great orator and his famous Gettysburg address still ranks high in terms of power and brevity. The sentences resonate today, especially the last bit: "that the nation, shall have a new birth of freedom, and that government of the people, by the people, for the people, shall not perish from the earth." He was also a great poetry lover. Here is one he wrote himself – in the autograph book of a hotel owner's daughter – he was staying there at the time, *To Rosa*:

> *You are young, and I am older;*
> *You are hopeful, I am not –*
> *Enjoy life, ere it grow colder –*
> *Pluck the roses ere they rot.*
> *Teach your beau to heed the lay –*
> *That sunshine soon is lost in shade –*
> *That now's as good as any day –*
> *To take thee, Rose, ere she fade.*
> *When I think of Lincoln's death or of anyone's untimely death, I always remember those simple lines of the great English poet John Donne: "any man's death diminishes me, because I am involved in mankind; and therefore never send to know for whom the bell tolls; it tolls for thee."*

Today I give thanks for great statesmen who put their country before themselves and their own safety.

November 7th

On this day in 1867 the Polish/French physicist and chemist Marie Curie was born. The only woman to have won a Nobel Prize twice, she coined the word 'radioactivity' and isolated the element Radium, which is the source of nuclear energy and x-rays.

She was known for her honesty and moderate life style and gave away much of her Nobel Prize money. Marie Curie seems to have been unaware, or indifferent to, the dangers that resulted from regular exposure to radiation.

She would often carry test tubes containing radio isotopes in her pocket. Her death from anaemia aged 66 was believed to be as a result of radiation exposure. There are not many poems written about medicine or atomic science, and fewer still that are good. Here is a poem by Robert Louis Stevenson who was troubled by illness for most of his life:

> *Fear not, dear friend, but freely live your days*
> *Though lesser lives should suffer. Such am I,*
> *A lesser life, that what is his of sky*
> *Gladly would give for you, and what of praise.*
> *Step, without trouble, down the sunlit ways.*
> *We that have touched your raiment, are made whole*
> *From all the selfish cankers of man's soul,*
> *And we would see you happy, dear, or die.*
> *Therefore be brave, and therefore, dear, be free;*
> *Try all things resolutely, till the best,*
> *Out of all lesser betters, you shall find;*
> *And we, who have learned greatness from you, we,*
> *Your lovers, with a still, contented mind,*
> *See you well anchored in some port of rest.*

Today I am grateful for the unselfish dreamers responsible for the demanding work that continues to be done in medical research.

November 8th

O n this day in 63 BC the famous Roman orator Marcus Tullius Cicero began his speeches against the conspirator Lucius Sergius Catilina. After the first speech, Catilina started plotting to have him murdered. In the often tarnished history of Rome, Cicero stands out as a truly great man, fearless in fighting for what he believed was right. In the chaos following the death of Julius Caesar, Cicero championed a return to traditional Republican government. He was eventually murdered in 43 BC. Today's poem is Shakespeare's magnificent paean to life well lived, from his play, *Cymbeline*:

> *Fear no more the heat o' the sun,*
> *Nor the furious winter's rages;*
> *Thou thy worldly task hast done,*
> *Home art gone, and ta'en thy wages:*
> *Golden lads and girls all must,*
> *As chimney-sweepers, come to dust.*
> *Fear no more the frown o' the great;*
> *Thou art past the tyrant's stroke;*
> *Care no more to clothe and eat;*
> *To thee the reed is as the oak:*
> *The scepter, learning, physic, must*
> *All follow this, and come to dust.*
> *Fear no more the lightning flash,*
> *Nor the all-dreaded thunder stone;*
> *Fear not slander, censure rash;*
> *Thou hast finished joy and moan:*
> *All lovers young, all lovers must*
> *Consign to thee, and come to dust.*
> *And renownèd be thy grave!*

Today I ask to do my best in all that I attempt, and to be true to myself.

November 9th

On this day in 1970 French soldier and statesman Charles de Gaulle died. Having served with distinction in World War I, de Gaulle's finest hour came in 1940 when he refused to accept the capitulation of France to the German invaders and led a small party of like-minded army officers to England to continue the struggle. For the next four years he rallied the French people via the BBC. Churchill and de Gaulle did not get on. Today's poem is about a different man at a different time, Don John of Austria, who was willing to stand up and fight when others would not, Lepanto by G K Chesterton. De Gaulle may have felt like Don John. He certainly felt like Joan of Arc and once told this to Churchill, who replied that the English "had to burn the last one." It starts:

> White founts falling in the courts of the sun,
> And the Soldan of Byzantium is smiling as they run;
> There is laughter like the fountains in that face of all men
> feared,
> It stirs the forest darkness, the darkness of his beard,
> It curls the blood-red crescent, the crescent of his lips,
> For the inmost sea of all the earth is shaken with his ships.
> They have dared the white republics up the capes of Italy,
> They have dashed the Adriatic round the Lion of the Sea,
> And the Pope has cast his arms abroad for agony and loss,
> And called the kings of Christendom for swords about the
> Cross,
> The cold queen of England is looking in the glass;
> The shadow of the Valois is yawning at the Mass;
> From evening isles fantastical rings faint the Spanish gun,
> And the Lord upon the Golden Horn is laughing in the sun.
> Strong gongs groaning as the guns boom far,
> Don John of Austria is going to the war

Today I give thanks for all brave men who put their country before their personal comfort.

November 10th

On this day in 1911 Andrew Carnegie formed his Carnegie Corporation for scholarly and charitable purposes. When he retired, he was one of the world's wealthiest men. He always had great respect for knowledge and education of any kind. He lived his life in three parts: learn, earn and return. He spent his early years learning and mastering the skills he needed, his middle life he spent accumulating huge sums of money and his later life he spent returning his fortune to the world as charitable donations. At the time of his death in 1919 aged 84, he had given away the equivalent of five billion dollars, at today's value. He never forgot his roots and in later years purchased and lived part of each year at Skibo Castle in the Highlands. Today's poem is a song of Scottish migrants remembering the old country, *Canadian Boat Song*:

> *From the lone shieling of the misty island*
> *Mountains divide us, and the waste of seas –*
> *Yet still the blood is strong, the heart is Highland,*
> *And we in dreams behold the Hebrides.*
> *We ne'er shall tread the fancy-haunted valley,*
> *Where 'tween the dark hills creeps the small clear stream,*
> *In arms around the patriarch banner rally,*
> *Nor see the moon on royal tombstones gleam.*
> *When the bold kindred, in the time long-vanish'd,*
> *Conquer'd the soil and fortified the keep, –*
> *No seer foretold the children would be banish'd,*
> *That a degenerate Lord might boast his sheep.*
> *Come foreign rage – let Discord burst in slaughter!*
> *O then for clansman true, and stern claymore –*
> *The hearts that would have given their blood like water,*
> *Beat heavily beyond the Atlantic roar.*

Today I give thanks for those that travel from one country to make a new life in another and by so doing, make the world a better place.

November 11th

On this day in 1821 the Russian novelist and writer Fyodor Dostoyevsky was born. In 1849 he was arrested for his involvement in the Petrashevsky Circle, a literary and political society. He was suspected of plotting revolution, and condemned to death. At the last moment, a note from Tsar Nicholas I was delivered to the firing squad, commuting the sentence to four years labour in Siberia. Dostoyevsky's addictions to gambling and beautiful women are well known. Here is part of a poem by Mikhail Lermontov, a poet that Dostoyevsky admired, *I'm to Believe*:

> I'm to believe, but with some fear,
> For I haven't tried it all before,
> That every monk could be sincere
> And live as he by altar swore;
> That smiles and kisses of all people
> Could be perfidious only once;
>
> That virtue is not just a sound,
> And life is more than a dream.
> But rough and hardened life's experience,
> Repulse my warm faith every time,
> My mind, sunk, as before, in grievance,
> Has not achieved its goal, prime,
> And heart, full of the sharp frustrations,
> Holds in its deep the clear trace
> Of dead – but blest imaginations,
> And vanished senses' easy shades;
> There will be none for it to fear,
> And what's a poison for all them,
> Makes it alive and feeds it here
> With its ironic, mocking flame.

Today I ask that I will be steadfast in my beliefs whatever the consequences may be.

November 12th

On this day in 1954, Ellis Island, located in New York harbour, the gateway to America, closed after processing more than 12 million immigrants since opening in 1892. On January 2, 1892, 15-year-old Annie Moore, from Ireland, became the first person to pass through the newly opened Ellis Island. She received a greeting from officials and a $10 gold piece. It was the largest sum of money she had ever had. Only two percent of immigrants were denied entrance into the U.S. Today, an estimated 40 percent of all Americans can trace their roots through Ellis Island. Less than two percent of Americans have indigenous roots. Today's poem is a sonnet which you will find engraved in bronze at the base of the Statue of Liberty. It was written by the American poet Emma Lazarus in 1883, to help raise funds for the erection of the statue, *The New Colossus*:

> *Not like the brazen giant of Greek fame,*
> *With conquering limbs astride from land to land;*
> *Here at our sea-washed, sunset gates shall stand*
> *A mighty woman with a torch, whose flame*
> *Is the imprisoned lightning, and her name*
> *Mother of Exiles. From her beacon-hand*
> *Glows world-wide welcome; her mild eyes command*
> *The air-bridged harbour that twin cities frame.*
> *"Keep, ancient lands, your storied pomp!" cries she*
> *With silent lips. "Give me your tired, your poor,*
> *Your huddled masses yearning to breathe free,*
> *The wretched refuse of your teeming shore.*
> *Send these, the homeless, tempest-tost to me,*
> *I lift my lamp beside the golden door!"*

Today I reflect on the welcome that America gave to immigrants while remembering the millions of indigenous Americans who suffered as a result through homelessness, death and disease.

November 13th

On this day in 1850 the Scottish writer Robert Louis Stevenson was born, creator of some of the most unforgettable characters in English literature: Long John Silver (modelled on a friend he fell out with) and Jim Hawkins from *Treasure Island*, Davy Balfour and Alan Breck from *Kidnapped* and the sinister split personality of *Dr Jekyll and Mr Hyde*. The grandson of the famous engineer Robert Stevenson, he was a strange and precocious child with a vivid imagination and a love of travel, which eventually took him to the Pacific Ocean with his wife Fanny. He settled and lived his last years on Samoa Island. It seems that he never lost the ability to see the world through the eyes of a child. In one story about him, he formally donated, by deed of gift, his own birthday to the daughter of an American Administrator on the Island, since she was born on Christmas Day and had no birthday celebration separate from the family's Christmas. Stevenson wrote some amazing poetry. Here is a beautiful poem called *Romance*:

> I will make you brooches and toys for your delight
> Of bird-song at morning and star-shine at night.
> I will make a palace fit for you and me
> Of green days in forests and blue days at sea.
> I will make my kitchen, and you shall keep your room,
> Where white flows the river and bright blows the broom,
> And you shall wash your linen and keep your body white
> In rainfall at morning and dewfall at night.
> And this shall be for music when no one else is near,
> The fine song for singing, the rare song to hear!
> That only I remember, that only you admire,
> Of the broad road that stretches and the roadside fire.

Today I give thanks for the genius of writers such as Stevenson; for the way they enrich our minds.

November 14th

On this day in 1851 the novel *Moby-Dick*, by Herman Melville was published. The book flopped, and it was many years before it was recognised as an American classic. Melville had been a sailor himself and had worked on whaling vessels in the Pacific. Moby-Dick is an enthralling read and the dangerous life of a 19th century whaler is fascinating enough, without the brooding and obsessive presence of the monomaniacal Captain Ahab, bent on wreaking vengeance on the great white mammal. Melville probably based his work on earlier accounts of an albino whale known as 'Mocha Dick' that had attacked several ships. It took him nearly two years to write the book that DH Lawrence called: "one of the strangest and most wonderful books in the world." Melville also wrote poetry. Here is a mournful example that might have been written by Ahab himself, *Dirge*:

> We drop our dead in the sea,
> The bottomless, bottomless sea;
> Each bubble a hollow sigh,
> As it sinks forever and aye.
> We drop our dead in the sea, –
> The dead reek not of aught;
> We drop our dead in the sea, –
> The sea ne'er gives it a thought.
> Sink, sink, oh corpse, still sink,
> Far down in the bottomless sea,
> Where the unknown forms do prowl,
> Down, down in the bottomless sea.
> 'Tis night above, and night all round,
> And night will it be with thee;
> As thou sinkest, and sinkest for aye,
> Deeper down in the bottomless sea.

Today I ask to be free of the corrosive effects of obsession and revenge.

November 15th

On this day in 1731 the English poet and writer of hymns William Cowper was born. Cowper changed 18th century poetry by writing about real people and things, and was a big influence on later romantic poets such as Coleridge and Wordsworth. He knew John Newton, who wrote the hymn Amazing Grace. Following a breakdown and time spent in an asylum for the insane, he experienced a spiritual awakening and wrote a number of beautiful hymns himself. Familiar phrases such as: "God moves in a mysterious way, His wonders to perform" and "Variety is the spice of life", are his. In his day, he was the most popular poet in the land. Here is a sonnet he wrote to Mary Unwin, a widow to whom he was greatly attached and who cared for him in difficult times, *To Mary Unwin*:

Mary! I want a lyre with other strings,
Such aid from Heaven as some have feign'd they drew,
An eloquence scarce given to mortals, new
And undebased by praise of meaner things;
That ere through age or woe I shed my wings,
I may record thy worth with honour due,
In verse as musical as thou art true,
And that immortalises whom it sings:
But thou hast little need. There is a Book
By seraphs writ with beams of heavenly light,
On which the eyes of God not rarely look,
A chronicle of actions just and bright –
  There all thy deeds, my faithful Mary, shine;
  And since thou own'st that praise, I spare thee mine.

Today I give thanks for the goodness and kindness that is found in people all over the world.

November 16th

On this day in 1950 the American doctor, Robert Smith, co-founder of Alcoholics Anonymous died aged 71. 'Dr Bob' was a chronic alcoholic who, until he met AA co-founder Bill Wilson in 1935, had tried every means he could to stop drinking, without success. The historic meeting of the two desperate men in a hotel room in Akron, Ohio laid the foundation of a world movement. Quite simply, they discovered that by being together and admitting their problems honestly and openly, they could stay sober. Today the movement is spread worldwide with an estimated membership of at least three million. Dr Bob and Bill W were two ordinary men who, together, turned their private hell into a salvation for millions. Dr Bob himself is estimated to have helped around five thousand alcoholics through personal interventions. It was not difficult to choose a suitable poem, *Invictus* by William Ernest Henley:

> Out of the night that covers me,
>   Black as the pit from pole to pole,
> I thank whatever gods may be
>   For my unconquerable soul.
> In the fell clutch of circumstance
>   I have not winced nor cried aloud.
> Under the bludgeonings of chance
>   My head is bloody, but unbowed.
> Beyond this place of wrath and tears
>   Looms but the Horror of the shade,
> And yet the menace of the years
>   Finds and shall find me unafraid.
> It matters not how strait the gate,
>   How charged with punishments the scroll,
> I am the master of my fate,
>   I am the captain of my soul.

Today I give thanks for the miracle of Alcoholics Anonymous and all other altruistic organisations.

November 17th

On this day in 1869 the Suez Canal opened to shipping. The canal is 100 miles long, of which 75 miles were excavated by an estimated 30 thousand workmen. An average of 50 ships per day pass through it. The canal was a great boost in the days of the British Empire, as ships travelling to India and the Eastern colonies no longer had to make the long trip round Africa via The Cape of Good Hope. They used to say that the sun never set on the British Empire but that's not the case today. Rudyard Kipling is called the poet of the British Empire. Here is his poem addressed to the USA, when their influence was increasing worldwide, *The White Man's Burden*:

> *Take up the White Man's burden –*
> *Send forth the best ye breed –*
> *Go send your sons to exile*
> *To serve your captives' need*
> *To wait in heavy harness*
> *On fluttered folk and wild –*
> *Your new-caught, sullen peoples,*
> *Half devil and half child*
>
> *Take up the White Man's burden –*
> *Have done with childish days –*
> *The lightly proffered laurel,*
> *The easy, ungrudged praise.*
> *Comes now, to search your manhood*
> *Through all the thankless years,*
> *Cold-edged with dear-bought wisdom,*
> *The judgment of your peers!*

Today I give thanks for the British Empire, for all its faults.

November 18th

On this day in 1991 Anglican Church envoy Terry Waite was released in Lebanon after more than four years in captivity in the hands of Islamic Jihadis.

Waite, the special envoy of the Archbishop of Canterbury, had earlier secured the release of several other hostages. The man who had once said, "Freeing hostages is like putting up a stage set, which you do with the captors, agreeing on each piece as you slowly put it together; then you leave an exit through which both the captor and the captive can walk with sincerity and dignity," had suddenly found himself playing a starring part in the drama.

During captivity, Waite said he was frequently blindfolded, beaten and subjected to mock executions. Since his release, Waite has been active in working for charitable causes and has written books about his experiences. "At the end of the day," he says, "love and compassion will win."

Today's poem is by Richard Lovelace, another man of principle who lived three hundred years before Terry Waite, *To Lucasta, on Going to the Wars*:

> *Tell me not, Sweet, I am unkind*
> * That from the nunnery*
> *Of thy chaste breast and quiet mind,*
> * To war and arms I fly.*
> *True, a new mistress now I chase,*
> * The first foe in the field;*
> *And with a stronger faith embrace*
> * A sword, a horse, a shield.*
> *Yet this inconstancy is such*
> * As you too shall adore;*
> *I could not love thee, Dear, so much,*
> * Loved I not Honour more.*

Today I give thanks for all brave men of principle, the world needs them.

November 19th

On this day in 1850 Alfred Tennyson became Poet Laureate succeeding William Wordsworth. The son of a country clergyman, Tennyson was the first to receive a peerage by virtue of his poetry. He remained Poet Laureate for 42 years and his work was highly popular in his lifetime. He met Queen Victoria, who recorded him in her diary as, "very peculiar looking, tall, dark, with a fine head, long black flowing hair & a beard, – oddly dressed, but there is no affectation about him". Tennyson's verse was influenced by the romantic poets, such as Wordsworth and Byron. He died in 1892 and is buried at Westminster Abbey. Here is my favourite Tennyson poem – *Crossing the Bar*:

> *Sunset and evening star,*
> *And one clear call for me!*
> *And may there be no moaning of the bar,*
> *When I put out to sea,*
> *But such a tide as moving seems asleep,*
> *Too full for sound and foam,*
> *When that which drew from out the boundless deep*
> *Turns again home.*
> *Twilight and evening bell,*
> *And after that the dark!*
> *And may there be no sadness of farewell,*
> *When I embark;*
> *For tho' from out our bourne of Time and Place*
> *The flood may bear me far,*
> *I hope to see my Pilot face to face*
> *When I have crost the bar.*

Today I give thanks for all the days that have been given to me and ask for courage to face the future, whatever it may hold.

November 20th

On this day in 1889 the American astronomer Edwin Hubble was born. A keen sportsman, Hubble saw combat duty in the First World War. He moved with his family to California, where he took part in the pioneering work at the observatories at Mount Wilson and Mount Palomar. At his death, no funeral was held for him, and his wife never revealed his burial site. The Hubble Space Telescope was launched into low Earth orbit in 1990 and still remains in operation. Its orbit outside the distortion of Earth's atmosphere allows it to take extremely high-resolution images with almost no background light, allowing a deep view into space and time. Many Hubble observations have led to breakthroughs in astrophysics, such as accurately determining the rate of expansion of the universe. Today's poem is the empowering and faith-filled poem by Gerard Manley Hopkins, *God's Grandeur*:

> *The world is charged with the grandeur of God.*
> *It will flame out, like shining from shook foil;*
> *It gathers to a greatness, like the ooze of oil*
> *Crushed. Why do men then now not reck his rod?*
> *Generations have trod, have trod, have trod;*
> *And all is seared with trade; bleared, smeared with toil;*
> *And wears man's smudge and shares man's smell: the soil*
> *Is bare now, nor can foot feel, being shod.*
> *And for all this, nature is never spent;*
> *There lives the dearest freshness deep down things;*
> *And though the last lights off the black West went*
> *Oh, morning, at the brown brink eastward, springs –*
> *Because the Holy Ghost over the bent*
> *World broods with warm breast and with ah! Bright wings.*

Today I give thanks for the grandeur of the universe and its vast unknown spaces. As Pascal said: "Le silence éternel de ces espaces infinis m'effraie" (The eternal silence of these infinite spaces terrifies me).

November 21st

On this day in 1694, François-Marie Arouet, later known as Voltaire, was born in Paris. He re-named himself Voltaire because he needed a pen name – he was always getting into trouble due to the scurrilous nature of his writings. In 1717 he spent almost a year in the Bastille for mocking the government.

Years later, in his novel Candide, Voltaire, in a reference to the real life execution of British Admiral Byng, for dereliction of duty, wrote "In this country, it is wise to kill an admiral from time to time to encourage the others." He would never have dared write anything similar in France. He lived in such fear of a backlash over his writings that he ended up living in Switzerland, just to be safe. He certainly played a part in starting the tidal wave of opinion that, 20 years after his death, became the French Revolution.

He wrote some delightful poetry. Here is a sample written at the age of 80, to a beautiful woman, *To Madame Lullin*:

> *Hey, what! You are amazed*
> *That after eighty winters*
> *My weak and antiquated muse*
> *Can still hum too?*
> *A bird may be heard*
> *After the season of sunny days;*
> *But his voice has nothing to reach;*
> *He no longer sings his love.*
> *So I touch my lyre again*
> *Which does not obey my fingers*
> *We are born, we live, shepherdess*
> *We die without knowing how:*
> *Everyone came out of nothing:*
> *Where does it go?*
> *God knows, my dear.*

Today I ask that I shall retain the ability to laugh and to keep trying, no matter what my age.

November 22nd

On this day in 1632 the English architect and astronomer Sir Christopher Wren was born. He will always be remembered as the architect of St Paul's, London's magnificent cathedral that was rebuilt after the great fire of 1666. Wren is buried there, and on the brass plaque that covers him are written these words, "Here in its foundations lies the architect of this church and city, Christopher Wren, who lived beyond 90 years, not for his own profit but for the public good. Reader, if you seek his monument – look around you". A notable scholar and astronomer, Wren also designed 52 other London churches after the fire as well as many other notable buildings. His architectural influence was immense and buildings such as the Pantheon in Paris and the Capitol in Washington DC were inspired by the dome of St Paul's. He seems to be a man who inspires a certain kind of clever poetry too. Here are two examples:

By Hugh Chesterman:

> "Clever men like Christopher Wren
> Only occur just now and then.
> No one expects, in perpetuity
> Architects of his ingenuity."

And by Edward Clerihew Bentley:

> "Sir Christopher Wren
> Said: 'I am going to dine with some men.
> If anyone calls: Say I am designing St. Paul's.'"

Today I give thanks for the beauty of some of our architecture.

November 23rd

On this day in 1963 US President John F Kennedy was assassinated in Dallas, Texas. Our knight in shining armour was taken from us. In fact, as later years revealed, Kennedy was no angel, as is true of many great men. The real Kennedy, as opposed to the celebrated hero promoted by his family, lacked true greatness because, while he had courage, he was deficient in integrity, compassion, and temperance. He was also a serial womaniser. "Dad told all the boys to get laid as often as possible," John Kennedy told a reporter, and "I can't get to sleep unless I've had a lay." Judging by the number of call girls, waitresses, office staff, actresses and other men's wives who claim to have 'known' him, he can have had few sleepless nights. What Kennedy did have however, was a capacity to inspire others to great things, and the thousand days of his presidency led the world to feel that they had a leader, at a time of fear and uncertainty. On this day in 1963 they lost that inspiration. Today's sonnet by Shakespeare, is about loss:

> Then hate me when thou wilt; if ever, now;
> Now, while the world is bent my deeds to cross,
> Join with the spite of fortune, make me bow,
> And do not drop in for an after-loss.
> Ah, do not, when my heart hath 'scaped this sorrow,
> Come in the rearward of a conquered woe;
> Give not a windy night a rainy morrow,
> To linger out a purposed overthrow.
> If thou wilt leave me, do not leave me last,
> When other petty griefs have done their spite,
> But in the onset come; so shall I taste
> At first the very worst of fortune's might,
> And other strains of woe, which now seem woe,
> Compared with loss of thee will not seem so.

Today I ask that our leaders be worthy of our trust and that they may carry out their duties safely.

November 24th

On this day in 1859 Charles Darwin published *On the Origin of Species by Means of Natural Selection*, a ground-breaking scientific work. Darwin's theory argued that organisms gradually evolve through a process he called "natural selection". Darwin's conclusions on evolution came to him during a five-year surveying expedition aboard HMS Beagle in the 1830s. However he was very reluctant to publish his findings because of his fear of the reaction from Christians – most of his theories go against bible teachings. When he did finally publish, over 20 years after the Beagle had returned to England, the book was a sensation. Darwin seems to have been a very single minded man who had little time for anything but his work. He once said: "I have tried lately to read Shakespeare, and found it so intolerably dull that it nauseates me." Today's poem has to be the opening lines of Vergil's Georgics, rendered by that master of English, John Dryden:

> *What makes a plenteous harvest, when to turn*
> *The fruitful soil, and when to sow the corn;*
> *The care of sheep, of oxen, and of kine,*
> *And how to raise on elms the teeming vine;*
> *The birth and genius of the frugal Bee,*
> *I sing, Maecenas, and I sing to thee.*
> *Ye deities! Who fields and plains protect,*
> *Who rule the seasons, and the year direct,*
> *Bacchus and fostering Ceres, powers divine,*
> *Who gave us corn for mast, for water, wine.*
> *Ye Fauns, propitious to the rural swains,*
> *Ye Nymphs, that haunt the mountains and the plains,*
> *Join in my work, and to my numbers bring*
> *Your needful succour; for your gifts I sing.*

Today I give thanks for the genius of great poets.

November 25th

On this day in 1970 the Japanese poet and writer Yukio Mishima committed ritual suicide. Considered one of the most important Japanese authors of the 20th century, he was nominated three times for the Nobel Prize for Literature. He is chiefly famous in the West for the manner of his death by suicide (seppuku) which he had apparently planned in advance. He and his companions had staged a coup on part of the military establishment, which they hoped would result in reinstatement of the Emperor; it did not work and had little effect. Mishima then stabbed himself in the stomach and was later beheaded by a close companion, as the ritual demanded. These lines were found by a man who committed suicide in a deep forest, in 1838:

> *Here, where the lonely hooting owl*
> *Sends forth his midnight moans,*
> *Fierce wolves shall o'er my carcase growl,*
> *Or buzzards pick my bones.*
> *No fellow-man shall learn my fate,*
> *Or where my ashes lie;*
> *Unless by beasts drawn round their bait,*
> *Or by the ravens' cry.*
> *Yes! I've resolved the deed to do,*
> *And this the place to do it:*
> *Sweet steel! Come forth from your sheath,*
> *And glist'ning, speak your powers;*
> *Rip up the organs of my breath,*
> *And draw my blood in showers!*
> *I strike! It quivers in that heart*
> *Which drives me to this end;*
> *I draw and kiss the bloody dart,*
> *My last – my only friend!*

Today I ask to be content with my lot and resist the urge to be overly dramatic or too famous, at the cost of my inner serenity.

November 26th

On this day in 1859 Charles Dickens published the last weekly instalment of *A Tale of Two Cities*. The book remains the best-selling novel of all time. Dickens pioneered the technique of writing by weekly instalments and thus was able to change and modify his stories if he received negative feedback (as for example, he once received from his wife's chiropodist). His stories were thus a form of early soap opera, and TV series today, such as *EastEnders*, owe a certain debt to Dickens. The realism in his stories was often drawn from personal experience, as he had a difficult childhood in poverty, his father being at times in a debtors' prison. Today's poem is by Dickens, though most people consider him a better novelist than a poet, *Lucy's Song*:

How beautiful at eventide
To see the twilight shadows pale,
Steal o'er the landscape, far and wide,
O'er stream and meadow, mound and dale!
How soft is Nature's calm repose
When ev'ning skies their cool dews weep:
The gentlest wind more gently blows,
As if to soothe her in her sleep!
The gay morn breaks,
Mists roll away,
All Nature awakes
To glorious day.
In my breast alone
Dark shadows remain;
The peace it has known
It can never regain.

Today I will do my best to ensure that the story of my life is a good one.

November 27th

On this day in 1914 Welsh poet Dylan Thomas was born. Now I know that they say he only wrote in English and that when he recited poems he sounded like an Englishman; I know they say he was a drunk and a womaniser and a spendthrift and a ne'er do well who borrowed from his friends and never paid them back. I know too that they say he could only write about childhood and death; it's probably all true, but when I read a poem like Fern Hill I'm moved by the lyrical beauty of the language and that's really all that matters. Certainly Dylan Thomas liked to drink and one wonders how much alcohol influenced his writing and his choice of words; it does seem that very few poets have been teetotal. Perhaps they need that loosening of inhibition that alcohol provides. CP Cavafy alludes to it in this poem, *Half an Hour*:

> I never had you, nor will I ever have you
> I suppose. A few words, an approach
> As in the bar yesterday, and nothing more.
> It is, undeniably, a pity. But we who serve Art
> Sometimes with intensity of mind, and of course only
> For a short while, we create pleasure
> Which almost seems real.
> So in the bar the day before yesterday – the merciful alcohol
> Was also helping much –
> I had a perfectly erotic half-hour.
> And it seems to me that you understood,
> And stayed somewhat longer on purpose.
> This was very necessary. Because
> For all the imagination and the wizard alcohol,
> I needed to see your lips as well,
> I needed to have your body close.

Today I give thanks for men of true genius who can turn a low mood into a happy one and give inspiration to so many.

November 28th

On this day in 1757 the English poet and painter William Blake was born. A lover of the Bible but hostile to the Church of England (indeed, to all forms of organised religion), Blake was influenced by the ideals and ambitions of the French and American Revolutions. He was considered beyond eccentric by many contemporaries for his idiosyncratic views and unconventional behaviour, but he is held in high regard by later critics for the force and creativity of his work. All his life he was a rebel against the misuse of power and a free thinker, but above all, he was a man of passion. Here is a Blake poem which is thought to express his advocacy of free love, *Earth's Answer*:

Earth raised up her head,
From the darkness dread & drear.
Her light fled:
Stony dread!
And her locks cover'd with grey despair.
Prison'd on watry shore
Starry Jealousy does keep my den
Cold and hoar
Weeping o'er
I hear the Father of the ancient men
Selfish father of men
Cruel, jealous, selfish fear
Can delight

Chain'd in night
The virgins of youth and morning bear.
Does spring hide its joy
When buds and blossoms grow?
Does the sower?
Sow by night?
Or the plowman in darkness plow?
Break this heavy chain,
That does freeze my bones around
Selfish! vain!
Eternal bane!
That free Love with bondage bound.

Today I give thanks for eccentric and passionate people who can lead us to reconsider our attitudes.

November 29th

On this day in 1935 the physicist Erwin Schrödinger published his famous thought experiment Schrödinger's Cat, a paradox that illustrates a problem of quantum mechanics. A cat, a flask of poison, and a radioactive source are placed in a sealed box. If an internal monitor detects radioactivity, the flask is shattered, releasing the poison that kills the cat. The Copenhagen interpretation of quantum mechanics implies that after a while, the cat is simultaneously alive and dead. Yet, when one looks in the box, one sees the cat either alive or dead, not both at once. This poses the question of when exactly quantum superposition ends and reality collapses into one possibility or the other. I hope that is all crystal clear. Schrödinger is reported to have said years later that he wished he had never thought of the wretched cat. Here is a poem about things not fully understood, *Brahma*, by Ralph Waldo Emerson:

> If the red slayer think he slays,
>   Or if the slain think he is slain,
> They know not well the subtle ways
>   I keep, and pass, and turn again.
> Far or forgot to me is near;
>   Shadow and sunlight are the same;
> The vanished gods to me appear;
>   And one to me are shame and fame.
> They reckon ill who leave me out;
>   When me they fly, I am the wings;
> I am the doubter and the doubt,
>   I am the hymn the Brahmin sings.
> The strong gods pine for my abode,
>   And pine in vain the sacred Seven;
> But thou, meek lover of the good!
>   Find me, and turn thy back on heaven.

Today I accept that there are things that I may not fully understand although I know that they may have value.

November 30th

On this day in 1874 Winston Churchill was born. Apart from being a hugely inspirational leader and a fearless warrior for his country he was also a gifted writer and speaker, a talented painter, and an accomplished bricklayer. I like this little verse he wrote in French, about his painting:

> *La peinture á l'huile*
> *Est bien difficile,*
> *Mais c'est beaucoup plus beau*
> *Que la peinture á l'eau.*

Churchill famously said: "I felt as if I were walking with destiny, and that all my past life had been but a preparation for this hour and for this trial . . . I thought I knew a good deal about it all, I was sure I should not fail." This poem by Ralph Waldo Emerson says the same thing:

> *Deep in the man sits fast his fate*
> *To mould his fortunes, mean or great:*
> *Unknown to Cromwell as to me*
> *Was Cromwell's measure or degree;*
> *Unknown to him as to his horse,*
> *If he than his groom be better or worse.*
> *He works, plots, fights, in rude affairs,*
> *With squires, lords, kings, his craft compares,*
> *Till late he learned, through doubt and fear,*
> *Broad England harbored not his peer:*
> *Obeying time, the last to own*
> *The Genius from its cloudy throne.*
> *For the prevision is allied*
> *Unto the thing so signified;*
> *Or say, the foresight that awaits*
> *Is the same Genius that creates.*

Today I reflect on the importance of accepting one's destiny.

December 1st

On this day in 1835 Hans Christian Andersen published his first book of fairy tales. Andersen lived in Denmark where he is now a 'national treasure'. Having had an unhappy and difficult childhood, Andersen found it virtually impossible to establish meaningful relationships with women and died alone; round his neck was a pouch containing a long letter from a childhood sweetheart towards whom his love had been unrequited. Though he died a rather lonely man, children and adults all over the world have reason to think kindly of him for the wonderful stories that he created. He wrote many poems, here is one example, *The Philosopher's Stone*:

> Life is a shadow that flits away
> In a night of darkness and woe.
> But then would follow brighter thoughts:
> Life has the rose's sweet perfume
> With sunshine, light, and joy.
> And if one stanza sounded painfully –
> Each mortal thinks of himself alone,
> Is a truth, alas, too clearly known;
> Then, on the other hand, came the answer –
> Love, like a mighty flowing stream,
> Fills every heart with its radiant gleam.
> She heard, indeed, such words as these –
> In the pretty turmoil here below,
> All is a vain and paltry show.
> In the blind girl's heart a stronger voice repeated –
> To trust in thyself and God is best,
> In His holy will forever to rest.
> But the evil spirit could not see this and remain contented.

Today I give thanks for those who through kindness and hard work contribute to the education and happiness of children.

December 2nd

On this day in 1804 Napoleon Bonaparte crowned himself Emperor of France. So much has been written about the man that there is little we don't know. Though usually described as small, he was, at 5ft 6 inches, about average height for world leaders – the same height as Churchill and Mussolini and one inch taller than Stalin and Margaret Thatcher.

Perhaps it is the comparison with pine tree Charles de Gaulle (6ft 5inches) that grates. Napoleon could handle huge armies but it seems that he couldn't handle women, as his wife Josephine had many lovers and indulged herself freely – her dress bill was bigger than that of Marie Antoinette. Napoleon's defeat at Waterloo was followed by six miserable years' exile on St Helena where he became increasingly frustrated and depressed; he was even said to have taken up gardening to pass the time.

His last words were: "France, army, head of the army, Joséphine." Many in England were sympathetic to Napoleon after his defeat, including Byron who wrote poems on the subject. Here is one, *Farewell to France*:

> Farewell to the Land, where the gloom of my glory
> Arose and o'ershadow'd the earth with her name –
> She abandons me now – but the page of her story,
> The brightest or blackest, is fill'd with my fame.

> Farewell to thee, France! – but when Liberty rallies

> Though withered, thy tears will unfold it again –
> Yet, yet I may baffle the hosts that surround us,
> And yet may thy heart leap awake to my voice –
> There are links which must break in the chain that has bound us
> Then turn thee and call on the Chief of thy choice!

Today I will reflect on the saying that 'pride comes before a fall' and ask that I will remain grateful for what I have.

December 3rd

O n this day in 1857 the novelist Józef Korzeniowski, later called Joseph Conrad, was born in Poland. Many of his stories tell of the struggles of the human spirit in times of adversity. His narrative style and anti-heroic characters have led to his categorisation as a modernist writer and he has influenced many others including Hemingway and Beckett.

Conrad's view of the world and our place in it seems almost Beckettian at times, as when he wrote: "In this world – as I have known it – we are made to suffer without the shadow of a reason, of a cause or of guilt . . . There is no morality, no knowledge and no hope; there is only the consciousness of ourselves which drives us about a world that is . . . but a clod of mud".

Today's poem is a different view of making do, by Lawrence Alma Tadema, *If No One Ever Marries Me*:

> *If no one ever marries me, –*
> *And I don't see why they should,*
> *For nurse says I'm not pretty,*
> *And I'm seldom very good –*
> *If no one ever marries me*
> *I shan't mind very much;*
> *I shall buy a squirrel in a cage,*
> *And a little rabbit-hutch:*
> *I shall have a cottage near a wood,*
> *And a pony all my own,*
> *And a little lamb quite clean and tame,*
> *That I can take to town:*
> *And when I'm getting really old, –*
> *At twenty-eight or nine –*
> *I shall buy a little orphan-girl*
> *And bring her up as mine.*

Today I give thanks for the strength of the human spirit that can overcome adversity through faith, hope and love.

December 4th

On this day in 1875 the Bohemian Austrian poet Rainer Maria Rilke was born. Rilke travelled a lot through Europe and eventually settled in Paris; he was part of the amazing artistic maelstrom that existed there in the first decade of the 20th century. His mystical and existential themes show him to be a modernist writer ahead of his time, but his poetry also contained great passion:

Extinguish my eyes, I'll go on seeing you.
Seal my ears, I'll go on hearing you
And without feet I can make my way to you.
Without a mouth I can swear your name

Sometimes it is almost metaphysical:

Do you remember still the falling stars
That like swift horses through the heavens raced
And suddenly leaped across the hurdles
Of our wishes – do you recall? And we
Did make so many! For there were countless numbers
Of stars: each time we looked above we were
Astounded by the swiftness of their daring play,
While in our hearts we felt safe and secure
Watching these brilliant bodies disintegrate,
Knowing somehow we had survived their fall.

Rilke died of leukaemia – he had already chosen his epitaph:

Rose, oh pure contradiction, delight
Of being no one's sleep under so
Many lids.

Today I am grateful for the mysticism and spirituality that give our existence a further dimension.

December 5th

On this day in 1791 Wolfgang Amadeus Mozart died. Experts debate to this day the possible causes of his death and whether it was from natural causes or something more sinister. Certainly Mozart said several times that he thought he had been poisoned.

Perhaps equally strange is the fact that so few people came to Mozart's funeral. He was after all possibly the greatest composer who ever lived. A few years before his death, Mozart had acquired a pet starling. He taught it to sing some bars of his music which he recorded in his notebook and was upset when it died. He carried out a mock burial and recited a poem he had composed for the occasion, *A Starling*:

> *Here lies a dear fool*
> *A little starling; in the prime*
> *Of his brief time.*
> *He must feel death's bitter pain.*
> *My heart is riven*
> *Thinking of him.*
> *Reader, shed a tear as well.*
> *He was not bad*
> *But frisky and bright.*
> *Underneath he was a wag,*
> *No one would deny;*
> *And I would say for sure*
> *That now he is above.*
> *In his friendly way*
> *He will be praising me.*
> *Yet unaware, I'd say*
> *That he's alive no more*
> *To thank me for this score.*

Today I will remember that we only have one life and we should make the best of it with whatever talents we have been given.

December 6th

On this day in 1877 Thomas A Edison made the first sound recording, reciting *Mary Had a Little Lamb* into his phonograph machine. Edison had been fascinated by science and nature since childhood. As an adult he became that rare thing, a brilliant scientist and a clever businessman. Among his inventions are the light bulb, the sound recorder and the movie camera. He also patented many industrial processes. He had a strong belief in a higher power in the universe saying: "I do not believe in the God of the theologians; but that there is a Supreme Intelligence I do not doubt." Non-violence was key to Edison's moral views. When asked to serve as a naval consultant for the First World War, he specified he would work only on defensive weapons saying later: "I am proud of the fact that I never invented weapons to kill." Today's poem is entitled *Discovery* by Edwin Arlington Robinson:

> We told of him as one who should have soared
> And seen for us the devastating light
> Whereof there is not either day or night,
> And shared with us the glamour of the Word
> That fell once upon Amos to record
> For men at ease in Zion, when the sight
> Of ills obscured aggrieved him and the might
> Of Hamath was a warning of the Lord.
> Assured somehow that he would make us wise,
> Our pleasure was to wait; and our surprise
> Was hard when we confessed the dry return
> Of his regret. For we were still to learn
> That earth has not a school where we may go
> For wisdom, or for more than we may know.

Today I give thanks for all discoveries that help mankind and ask for wisdom in their use.

December 7th

On this day in 1985 the English writer and poet Robert Graves died aged 90. Graves was a classical scholar and his historical novels *I Claudius* and *Claudius the God* about the decadence and intrigues of the Roman Empire, were hugely successful; his study of poetic inspiration, *The White Goddess*, has never been out of print.

His interpretations of the Greek myths were also well received. An expert on the classical world, he was given to conversing with his learned friends in Latin. He was also a noted poet and literary critic and his poetry of the First World War (he was severely wounded in France) is particularly fine. Graves lived for many years in Majorca and is buried there after his death aged 90.

Here is a poem by German Mathias Claudius, Der Tod und das Mädchen (Death and the Maiden):

The Maiden:

> *"It's all over! Alas, it's all over now!*
> *Go, savage man of bone!*
> *I am still young – go, devoted one!*
> *And do not molest me."*
> *Death:*
> *"Give me your hand, you fair and tender form!*
> *I am a friend; I do not come to punish.*
> *Be of good cheer! I am not savage.*
> *You shall sleep gently in my arms."*

Today I will try to 'wear the world like a loose garment' and be glad to show my feelings so that others may see my true self.

December 8th

On this day in 65 BC the Roman poet Quintus Horatius Flaccus was born. Affectionately known by classicists as Horace, he is loved for his enchanting lyric poetry but also for his self-deprecatory view on life (not a common Roman attitude).

He fought in the Battle of Philippi but ran away, he tells us that he prefers to have a nap than write poetry and complains of waiting up half the night for a girlfriend who never comes. In short, he is human. A friend of Vergil, he wrote about people and love.

Here is an ode by Horace, translated by AE Housman who called it "the most beautiful poem in ancient literature": *Diffugere Nives*:

> The snows are fled away, leaves on the shaws
> And grasses in the mead renew their birth,
> The river to the river-bed withdraws,
> And altered is the fashion of the earth.
> The Nymphs and Graces three put off their fear
> And unapparelled in the woodland play.
> The swift hour and the brief prime of the year
> Say to the soul, Thou wast not born for aye.
> Thaw follows frost; hard on the heel of spring
> Treads summer sure to die, for hard on hers
> Comes autumn with his apples scattering;
> Then back to wintertide, when nothing stirs.
>
> Come we where Tullus and where Ancus are
> And good Aeneas, we are dust and dreams.
> Torquatus, if the gods in heaven shall add
> The morrow to the day, what tongue has told?
> Feast then thy heart, for what thy heart has had
> The fingers of no heir will ever hold.

Today I give thanks for being alive and for being able to see and enjoy the seasons of the year as they come and go.

December 9th

On this day in 1608 the English poet John Milton was born, 16 years before the death of Shakespeare. His Republican views brought him into favour with Cromwell but after the return of the monarchy, he faded into obscurity and died in relative poverty in 1674 at the age of 65. A scholar with a command of several languages, he was appointed Secretary for Foreign Tongues in 1649. He is noted for his morality and piety rather than for romanticism or humour. By 1654 he was completely blind and much of his work was produced through dictation, mostly to his daughters who described him as being in the mornings like 'a cow ready for milking', pacing the room until he had been unburdened of his verse. Though somewhat out of fashion nowadays, his poetry is very fine. Here is that poignant sonnet *On His Blindness*:

> *When I consider how my light is spent,*
> *Ere half my days, in this dark world and wide,*
> *And that one Talent which is death to hide*
> *Lodged with me useless, though my Soul more bent*
> *To serve therewith my Maker, and present*
> *My true account, lest he returning chide;*
> *"Doth God exact day-labour, light denied?"*
> *I fondly ask. But patience, to prevent*
> *That murmur, soon replies, "God doth not need*
> *Either man's work or his own gifts; who best*
> *Bear his mild yoke, they serve him best. His state*
> *Is Kingly. Thousands at his bidding speed*
> *And post o'er Land and Ocean without rest:*
> *They also serve who only stand and wait."*

Today I give thanks for the talents that I have and ask that I may use them to the best of my ability and not be disheartened by setbacks.

December 10th

On this day in 1830 the American writer and poet Emily Dickinson was born. Eccentric and reclusive, with a penchant for white clothing, she spent much of her adult life inside the large family home at Amherst in Massachusetts, often not leaving her room for days on end.

Thomas Higginson, a literary critic and ex-minister gave her considerable moral support but only met her once. He left this telling description: "A little plain woman with two smooth bands of reddish hair in a very plain and exquisitely clean white piqué and a blue net worsted shawl." He also felt that he never met "with anyone who drained my nerve power so much. Without touching her, she drew from me. I am glad not to live near her."

Here is one of her strange poems: *Why do I love You, Sir?*

Because –
The Wind does not require the Grass
To answer – wherefore when He pass
She cannot keep Her place.
Because He knows –
Do not You –
And We know not –
Enough for Us
The Wisdom it be so –
The Lightning – never asked an Eye
Wherefore it shut – when He was by –
Because He knows it cannot speak –
And reasons not contained –
Of Talk –
There be – preferred by Daintier Folk –
The Sunrise – Sire – compelleth Me –
Because He's Sunrise – and I see –
Therefore – Then – I love Thee –

Today I reflect on people's individuality and the need not to judge others.

December 11th

On this day in 1918 the Russian writer Aleksandr Solzhenitsyn was born. Soon after the war he was arrested for disparaging remarks made about Stalin and sentenced to eight years in a prison camp. This was followed by lengthy exile in Kazakhstan, where he was diagnosed with cancer.

All this provided first hand material for his books, especially *One Day in the Life of Ivan Denisovich* and *Cancer Ward*. His writing is notable for its brutal realism and the underlying strength of the human spirit that it describes; the emotion in describing a prisoner's joy at finding a piece of cabbage in his watery soup for example, is quite unique. Today's poem was written by another man who spent time in jail, Oscar Wilde. Here are the last verses of *The Ballad Of Reading Gaol*:

> In Reading gaol by Reading town
> There is a pit of shame,
> And in it lies a wretched man
> Eaten by teeth of flame,
> In a burning winding-sheet he lies,
> And his grave has got no name.
> And there, till Christ call forth the dead,
> In silence let him lie:
> The man had killed the thing he loved,
> And so he had to die.
> And all men kill the thing they love,
> By all let this be heard,
> Some do it with a bitter look,
> Some with a flattering word,
> The coward does it with a kiss,
> The brave man with a sword!

Today I ask that I may remain steadfast and strong in my journey along the road of life.

December 12th

On this day in 1821 the French writer Gustave Flaubert was born. His reputation really comes from Madame Bovary, his amazing debut novel that tells a basically simple tale of a provincial wife's infidelity. What makes the book so special is the way Flaubert balances the realism of the story with the nuances of each character's fears and aspirations.

Consider poor deluded Emma Bovary, a caged bird, trapped and frustrated in her humdrum life: "Though she had no one to write to, she had bought herself a blotter, a writing case, a pen and envelopes; she would dust off her whatnot, look at herself in the mirror, take up a book, and then begin to daydream and let it fall to her lap . . . She wanted to die. And she also wanted to live in Paris."

Today's poem is by Paul Laurence Dunbar, entitled Sympathy, about another caged bird:

> I know what the caged bird feels, alas!
>   When the sun is bright on the upland slopes;
> When the wind stirs soft through the springing grass,
> And the river flows like a stream of glass;
>   When the first bird sings and the first bud opes,
> And the faint perfume from its chalice steals –
> I know what the caged bird feels!
> I know why the caged bird beats his wing
>   Till its blood is red on the cruel bars;
> When his wing is bruised and his bosom sore, –
> When he beats his bars and he would be free;
> It is not a carol of joy or glee,
>   But a prayer that he sends from his heart's deep core,
> But a plea, that upward to Heaven he flings –
> I know why the caged bird sings!

Today I ask that I be motivated by my real needs and thoughts rather than by my delusions, fears and aspirations.

December 13th

On this day in 1797 the German poet Heinrich Heine was born in Dusseldorf. Heine's early lyrical poetry was well received and often set to music by, amongst others, Haydn and Schubert. Later on he moved to Paris and distanced himself from Romanticism by adding irony and satire into his poetry, sometimes mocking the sentimental-romantic awe of nature in the work of his contemporaries. In Paris, Heine became friends with Karl Marx and shared some of his views. Many years later his work was banned by the Nazis. Some of his writing seems oddly prophetic: "A play will be performed in Germany which will make the French Revolution look like an innocent idyll." And "Where books are burned, then in the end people will be burned too". Here is one of his best known poems from his lyrical period, *Lorelei*:

I don't know what it could mean,
Or why I'm so sad: I find,
A fairy-tale, from times unseen,
Won't vanish from my mind.
The air is cool and it darkens,
And quiet flows the Rhine:
The tops of the mountains sparkle,
In evening's after-shine.
The loveliest of maidens,
She's wonderful, sits there,
Her golden jewels glisten,
She combs her golden hair.
She combs it with a comb of gold,
And sings a song as well:
Its strangeness too is old
And casts a powerful spell.
It grips the boatman in his boat
With a wild pang of woe:
He only looks up to the heights,
Can't see the rocks below.
The waves end by swallowing
The boat and its boatman,
That's what, by her singing,
The Lorelei has done.

Today I ask that I am steadfast in pursuing my goals in life and not be lured from them by the Lorelei of instant gratification.

December 14th

On this day in 1799 the greatest American statesman George Washington died, 'First in war, first in peace and first in the hearts of his countrymen'. In France, Napoleon declared ten days of mourning – Washington had after all, shown the French how to do revolution. A man of great physical strength, his favourite sport was fox-hunting. He had trouble with his teeth from an early age and had several sets of false teeth made but was often in pain from toothache – some of this distress is said to be evident in portraits, including the likeness on the one dollar bill. Today's poem is an oddity – a sonnet that was written in 1936 by David Shulman. Perhaps not the greatest in style, it is an anagrammatic poem – in this case, a 14-line rhyming sonnet, in which every line is an anagram of the title. An extraordinary work about an extraordinary man, *Washington Crossing the Delaware*:

> A hard, howling, tossing water scene.
> Strong tide was washing hero clean.
> "How cold!" Weather stings as in anger.
> O Silent night shows war ace danger!
> The cold waters swashing on in rage.
> Redcoats warn slow his hint engage.
> When star general's action wish'd "Go!"
> He saw his ragged continentals row.
> Ah, he stands – sailor crew went going.
> And so this general watches rowing.
> He hastens – winter again grows cold.
> A wet crew gain Hessian stronghold.
> George can't lose war with's hands in;
> He's astern – so go alight, crew, and win!

Today I ask that I may learn from the power of example shown by upright men and women and that I too may be an example to others.

December 15th

On this day in AD 37 the Roman Emperor Nero Claudius Caesar was born. The last of the Julio Claudian emperors, a dynasty that mainly received a negative press at the hands of contemporary historians Suetonius and Tacitus, Nero is famous for fiddling while Rome burned and then blaming the fire on the Christians. He also had his mother executed and probably poisoned his stepbrother.

But he was popular with the common people, and during his reign the empire increased in size and strength. When Galba, the governor of the Spanish province, was said to be making a bid for the throne, Nero committed suicide, wrongly thinking that he was about to be deposed and assassinated. Perhaps a fitting end for a man that early Christians at the time considered to be 'The Antichrist'. Here is a poem on Nero's death by CF Cavafy, *Nero's Dilemma*:

> Nero wasn't worried at all when he heard
> The utterance of the Delphic Oracle:
> "Beware the age of seventy-three."
> Plenty of time to enjoy himself still.
> He's thirty. The deadline
> The god has given him is quite enough
> To cope with future dangers.
> Now, a little tired, he'll return to Rome –
> But wonderfully tired from that journey
> Devoted entirely to pleasure:
> Theatres, garden-parties, stadiums . . .
> Evenings in the cities of Achaia . . .
> So much for Nero. And in Spain Galba
> Secretly musters and drills his army –
> Galba, the old man in his seventy-third year.

Today I ask that I will never give in to despair and to see setbacks as opportunities.

December 16th

O n this day in 1770 the German composer and musician Ludwig van Beethoven was born. He is said to have met Mozart once in Vienna when Beethoven, then aged 16, came to visit. Mozart was in a bad mood and did not relish having to stop work to listen to a young prodigy. "Play something," he told Beethoven. Beethoven played the opening of Mozart's *C minor Piano Concerto*. "Not that," said Mozart. "Anybody can play that. Play something of your own." Beethoven did. Whereupon Mozart called to his wife Constanze: "Stanzi, Stanzi, watch out for that boy. One day he will give the world something to talk about." Beethoven died aged 56, almost totally deaf, of complications that may have been alcohol related. My poem today is Emily Dickinson's strange *Better Than Music*:

Better – than Music! For I – who heard it –
I was used – to the Birds – before –
This – was different –'Twas Translation –
Of all tunes I knew – and more –
'Twasn't contained – like other stanza –
No one could play it – the second time –
But the Composer – perfect Mozart –
Perish with him – that Keyless Rhyme!
So – Children – told how Brooks in Eden –
Bubbled a better – Melody –

Not such a strain – the Church – baptizes –
When the last Saint – goes up the Aisles –
Not such a stanza splits the silence –
When the Redemption strikes her Bells –
Let me not spill – its smallest cadence –
Humming – for promise – when alone –
Humming – until my faint Rehearsal –
Drop into tune – around the Throne –

Today I give thanks for geniuses like Beethoven.

December 17th

On this day in 1807 The American Quaker poet and anti-slavery campaigner John Greenleaf Whittier was born. His poetry was well received during his lifetime and he was a friend of Longfellow and Emerson. Here is Whittier's poem about the ancient oriental drug, Soma. This is also the name of a fictional drug in Aldous Huxley's 1932 novel, *Brave New World*. It is described as "All of the benefits of Christianity and alcohol without their defects." Not, I think, how Whittier would have seen it:

> The fagots blazed, the caldron's smoke
> Up through the green wood curled;
> "Bring honey from the hollow oak,
> Bring milky sap," the brewers spoke,
> In the childhood of the world.
> And brewed they well or brewed they ill,
> The priests thrust in their rods,
> First tasted, and then drank their fill,
> And shouted, with one voice and will,
> "Behold the drink of gods!"
> They drank, and lo! in heart and brain
> A new, glad life began;
> The gray of hair grew young again,
> The sick man laughed away his pain,
> The cripple leaped and ran
>
> And yet the past comes round again,
> And new doth old fulfil;
> In sensual transports wild as vain
> We brew in many a Christian fane
> The heathen Soma still!

Today I ask to live free of addiction from mood altering substances of any kind.

December 18th

On this day in 1879 the Swiss born German artist Paul Klee was born. Highly influential at a time of great changes in the art world, Klee and his friend Wassily Kandinsky were teaching colleagues at the celebrated Bauhaus school. Klee wrote books on art theory, particularly colour, and gave many lectures. His enquiring mind and readiness to experiment with colour and form, in 'taking a line for a walk', endeared him to many of the modernist painters. He also wrote some interesting poetry:

> In the beginning there was . . . ?
> Things moved freely,
> So to speak, neither in a curve
> Nor in a straight line. Think of them
> As moving elementally, they go
> Wherever they go, in order to go
> Destination-less intent-less disobedient
> With movement the only certainty,
> A "state" of elemental motion.
> It is at first only a principle: to move,
> Not a movement principle,
> No particular intent,
> Nothing special, nothing organised.
> Chaos and anarchy, murky seething
> Intangible, nothing heavy nothing
> Light (heavy-light) nothing white
> Nothing black nothing white (only greyish) nothing red nothing
>   yellow
> Nothing blue (only greyish) not even directly grey, nothing at all
> Distinct only indeterminate, vague

Today I give thanks for an enquiring mind and ask that it remains that way.

December 19th

On this day in 1848 Emily Brontë, author of *Wuthering Heights*, died at the tragically early age of 30. The most reclusive of the Brontë sisters, Emily seems to have had few friends and indeed spoke to few people outside her family; many thought her book had been written by a man. It was her only novel. How she managed to write a work of such passion and emotion while living in seclusion, it is hard to imagine. Emily wrote poetry too, but today's offering are the sad and moving lines that her sister Charlotte wrote on losing her, *On the Death of Emily Jane Brontë*:

> *My darling thou wilt never know*
> *The grinding agony of woe*
> *That we have bourne for thee,*
> *Thus may we consolation tear*
> *E'en from the depth of our despair*
> *And wasting misery.*
> *The nightly anguish thou art spared*
> *When all the crushing truth is bared*
> *To the awakening mind,*
> *When the galled heart is pierced with grief,*
> *Till wildly it implores relief,*
> *But small relief can find.*
> *Nor know'st thou what it is to lie*
> *Looking forth with streaming eye*
> *On life's lone wilderness*
> *Then since thou art spared such pain*
> *We will not wish thee here again;*
> *He that lives must mourn.*
> *God help us through our misery*
> *And give us rest and joy with thee*
> *When we reach our bourne!*

Today I give thanks for all great writers and seek to appreciate how the emotions of real life can be expressed in written form.

December 20th

On this day in 1192 King Richard the Lionheart, on his way home from the Crusades, was captured and imprisoned by Duke Leopold of Austria on the outskirts of Vienna. In spite of the danger of capture and ransom, he had tried to hurry home overland rather than by ship, travelling in disguise with a small band of companions.

The story goes that it was his demands for roast chicken rather than humbler fare at the inn where he stayed that aroused suspicion. He was eventually ransomed in 1194 for the huge sum of 150,000 marks. This required an extraordinary tax raising exercise in England – churches were forced to give up valuables, monasteries had to turn over a season's wool harvest, and everyone had to contribute. If the phrase 'a king's ransom' was not known at the time, it was probably invented then.

One calls to mind that old French marching song, Auprès de ma blonde which mentions ransom of a kind:

Dites-nous Donc ma belle	*"Tell us, my pretty girl*
Où est votre Mari?	*Where is your husband?"*
Il est dans la Hollande,	*"He is in Holland –*
les Hollandais l'ont pris.	*The Dutch have captured him."*
Que donneriez vous belle	*"What would you give my pretty,*
Pour revoir votre Mari?	*To see him again?"*
Je donnerai Versailles,	*"Oh I would give Versailles,*
Paris et Saint Denis.	*Paris and Saint Denis."*
Auprès de ma blonde	*Auprès de ma blonde etc.*
Qu'il fait bon, fait bon, fait bon	

We always want our loved ones back and King Richard was well loved. His ransom money was roughly equivalent to the normal total of taxes raised in a year in England. Somehow they found it.

Today I give thanks for all those who are prepared to show their love for others in practical ways.

December 21st

On this day on 1841 the New Zealand poet and writer Thomas Bracken was born. Bracken emigrated from Ireland aged 12 and did a number of jobs before becoming a successful journalist. He was also for a time a Member of Parliament and a champion of the Maori people. His poetry soon became noticed and he composed one version of the country's national anthem, 'God Defend New Zealand'.

Here is part of one of his poems, *Not Understood* – I think it is rather fine:

> *Not understood, we move along asunder;*
> *Our paths grow wider as the seasons creep*
> *Along the years; we marvel and we wonder*
> *Why life is life, and then we fall asleep*
> *Not understood.*
> *Not understood, we gather false impressions*
> *And hug them closer as the years go by;*
> *Till virtues often seem to us transgressions;*
> *And thus men rise and fall, and live and die*
> *Not understood.*
> *Not understood! Poor souls with stunted vision*
> *Oft measure giants with their narrow gauge;*
> *The poisoned shafts of falsehood and derision*
> *Are oft impelled 'gainst those who mould the age,*
> *Not understood.*
> *Not understood! The secret springs of action*
> *I am come again.*

Today I ask for tolerance for the shortcomings of others and the recognition that true love includes patience and forgiveness.

December 22nd

On this day in 1869 the poet Edwin Arlington Robinson was born in Maine. Robinson published his first work while at Harvard where he seems to have set his sights low.

He left after two years following the death of his father. At the age of 24 he wrote: "Writing has been my dream ever since I was old enough to lay a plan for an air castle." Gradually his work gained recognition and in his lifetime he won three Pulitzer Prizes.

Here is part of his early poem, *Ballad of a Ship*:

> *Down by the flash of the restless water*
> *The dim White Ship like a white bird lay;*
> *Laughing at life and the world they sought her,*
> *And out she swung to the silvering bay.*
> *Then off they flew on their roistering way,*
> *And the keen moon fired the light foam flying*
> *Up from the flood where the faint stars play,*
> *And the bones of the brave in the wave are lying.*
> *'T was a king's fair son with a king's fair daughter,*
> *And full three hundred beside, they say,*
> *Revelling on for the lone, cold slaughter*
> *So soon to seize them and hide them for aye;*
> *But they danced and they drank and their souls grew gay,*
> *Nor ever they knew of a ghoul's eye spying*
> *Through the mist of a drunken dream they brought her*
> *(This wild white bird) for the sea-fiend's prey:*
> *The pitiless reef in his hard clutch caught her,*
> *And hurled her down where the dead men stay.*
> *A torturing silence of wan dismay –*
> *Shrieks and curses of mad souls dying –*
> *Then down they sank to slumber and sway*
> *Where the bones of the brave in the wave are lying.*

Today I will reflect that small steps are sometimes the best.

December 23rd

On this day in 1894 Claude Debussy's *Prélude à l'après-midi d'un faune* was first performed in Paris. Based on French poet Stéphane Mallarmé's beautiful poem, the work was well received.

He was a child prodigy and a brilliant pianist as well as a composer. It was a different story, though, in 1912 when the Ballets Russes of Diaghilev gave their first performance of the work in dance form. The brilliant but erotic dancing of the star male dancer, Nijinsky, was too much for the audience – on the second night the police were called.

Debussy's private life was chaotic and, though twice married, he had numerous affairs. He stayed briefly at Eastbourne when things got too difficult at home and during his stay wrote his famous piece La mer.

Here is the beginning of Stéphane Mallarmé's poem that had inspired him, The Afternoon of a Faun:

These nymphs, I would perpetuate them. So bright
Their crimson flesh that hovers there, light
In the air drowsy with dense slumbers.
Did I love a dream?
My doubt, mass of ancient night, ends extreme
In many a subtle branch, that remaining the true
Woods themselves, proves, alas, that I too
Offered myself, alone, as triumph, the false ideal of roses.
Let's see . . .
or if those women you note
Reflect your fabulous senses' desire!
Faun, illusion escapes from the blue eye,
Cold, like a fount of tears, of the most chaste:
But the other, she, all sighs, and contrasts you say
Like a breeze of day warm on your fleece?

Today I ask for the ability to see new meanings in life and to pass on to others the chance to re-evaluate their own visions.

December 24th

On this day in 1818 Franz Gruber, a teacher and organist in Arnsdorf, Austria, composed the music of the Christmas carol *Silent Night*. In Britain, the carol tradition began in the 15th century and by the 19th century was highly popular entertainment.

Since much of church services in the Middle Ages was in Latin, carols were a way of getting the Christmas message across to the common people. The Victorians were the ones to glamourise Christmas with the introduction of the tree and Christmas cards. Charles Dickens wrote *A Christmas Carol* in 1843 which was an instant success.

Here is Gruber's carol:

> *Silent night! Holy night!*
> *All is calm all is bright*
> *Round yon virgin mother and child*
> *Holy infant so tender and mild*
> *Sleep in heavenly peace!*
> *Sleep in heavenly peace*
> *Silent night! Holy night!*
> *Son of God love's pure light*
> *Radiant beams from thy holy face*
> *With the dawn of redeeming grace,*
> *Jesus, Lord at thy birth*
> *Jesus, Lord at thy birth*
> *Silent night! Holy night!*
> *Shepherds quake at the sight*
> *Glories stream from heaven afar*
> *Heavenly hosts sing Alleluia*
> *Christ the Saviour is born*
> *Christ the Saviour is born*

Today I give thanks for my existence and for that of the whole world; I ask that those I love will find their own spiritual experiences and that the blessings of peace may be upon us all.

December 25th

Today people all over the world celebrate the birth of Jesus Christ. Purists have long argued over the exact date that this happened. About the only agreement they have is that it was not on December 25th. Does it matter?

The world seems to stop and take a breath every Christmas day as if to say "Let's all be calm and peaceful for once" and usually it works – for the day. Perhaps we have to be thankful for just that. At Christmas in 1864, Henry Wadsworth Longfellow received news that his son had been seriously wounded in the American Civil War. He wrote this:

I heard the bells on Christmas day
Their old familiar carols play,
And wild and sweet,
The words repeat
Of peace on earth, good will to men.
I thought how, as the day had come,
The belfries of all Christendom
Had rolled along
The unbroken song
Of peace on earth, good will to men.
Till ringing, singing, on its way,
The world revolved from night to day,
A voice, a chime
A chant sublime
Of peace on earth good will to men.
Then from each black, accursed mouth

The cannon thundered in
* the south*
And with the sound
The carols drowned
Of peace on earth good
* will to men.*
Then pealed the bells more
* loud and deep:*
"God is not dead, nor doth
* He sleep;*
The wrong shall fail,
The right prevail
With peace on earth,
* good will to men."*

Today I give thanks to my higher power and remember that Christmas is about giving and receiving.

December 26th

On this day in 1947 the play *The Glass Menagerie* by Tennessee Williams was premiered in New York. Williams did not write this, his first play until he was 34. It has been called one of the greatest American dramas ever written and like most of his work, it was drawn from experience within his own highly dysfunctional family.

His father was an alcoholic, his mother went mad and his sister was given a lobotomy. Williams himself struggled with his homosexuality and his lifestyle became a drink and drugs fuelled rampage. Yet for a few years while he produced *A Streetcar Named Desire*, *Suddenly Last Summer* and *Cat on a Hot Tin Roof*, he was the world's most famous playwright.

Perhaps surprisingly, the man whose violent and emotional lifestyle matched his work and who once said "Don't look forward to the day you stop suffering, because when it comes you'll know you're dead," lived to the age of 72. His great plays live on and are still regularly performed.

Today's poem, *Night*, by Francis William Bourdillon, is about love:

> The night has a thousand eyes,
> And the day but one;
> Yet the light of the bright world dies
> With the dying sun.
>
> The mind has a thousand eyes,
> And the heart but one;
> Yet the light of a whole life dies,
> When love is done.

Today I will try to live my life with passion of a positive kind and try to understand the passions of other people.

December 27th

On this day in 1983 Pope John Paul II met Mehmet Ali Ağca, the man who had shot him two years previously in an attempt to kill him. The attack happened as the Pope was shaking hands and lifting small children in his arms while being driven around St Peter's square.

Suddenly, there was a burst of gunfire – four shots were fired and the Pope faltered and fell into the arms of his Polish secretary, who was in the car with him. Following the shooting, the Pope asked people to pray for Ağca "whom I have sincerely forgiven."

He and Ağca met and spoke privately at the prison where Ağca was being held and a friendship is said to have developed. In early February 2005, during the Pope's illness, he sent a letter to the Pope wishing him well. Ağca gave several reasons for the shooting, but it seems possible that it was instigated by the Soviet Union because of the Solidarity uprisings in Poland.

Today's poem is really a hymn about forgiveness by John Donne, *A Hymn to God the Father*:

> *Wilt thou forgive that sin where I begun,*
> *Which was my sin, though it were done before?*
> *Wilt thou forgive that sin, through which I run,*
> *And do run still, though still I do deplore?*
> *When thou hast done, thou hast not done,*
> *For I have more.*
> *I have a sin of fear, that when I have spun*
> *My last thread, I shall perish on the shore;*
> *But swear by thyself, that at my death thy Son*
> *Shall shine as he shines now, and heretofore;*
> *And, having done that, thou hast done;*
> *For I fear no more.*

Today I ask that I be not too proud or angry to recognise when I have done wrong and to ask for forgiveness.

December 28th

On this day in AD 1 it is said that King Herod of Judea ordered the massacre of all children under the age of two in the neighbourhood of Bethlehem. His plan was to eliminate any possible emergence of a Messiah who might challenge his authority. As the scriptures tell it; "An angel of the Lord appeared to Joseph in a dream. Get up, he said, take the child and his mother and escape to Egypt. Stay there until I tell you, for Herod is going to search for the child to kill him. So he got up, took the child and his mother during the night and left for Egypt, where he stayed until the death of Herod". When Herod realised that he had been outwitted, he was furious, and he gave orders to kill all the boys in Bethlehem and its vicinity. Thus the prophecy of Jeremiah was fulfilled: "A voice is heard in Ramah, weeping and great mourning, Rachel weeping for her children." Here is Oscar Wilde's Sonnet about a more recent massacre – *The Slaughter of the Christians in Bulgaria*:

> Christ, dost thou live indeed? or are thy bones
> Still straightened in their rock-hewn sepulchre?
> And was thy Rising only dreamed by Her
> Whose love of thee for all her sin atones?
> For here the air is horrid with men's groans,
> The priests who call upon thy name are slain,
> Dost thou not hear the bitter wail of pain
>
> From those whose children lie upon the stones?
> Come down, O Son of God! incestuous gloom
> Curtains the land, and through the starless night
> Over thy Cross the Crescent moon I see!
> If thou in very truth didst burst the tomb
> Come down, O Son of Man! and show thy might,
> Lest Mahomet be crowned instead of Thee!

Today I give thanks for the birth and life of Christ. I ask that slaughter and suffering in the world will cease.

December 29th

On this day in 1170 Thomas Beckett, Archbishop of Canterbury, was murdered in his cathedral by followers of King Henry II of England. It was the culmination of years of legal and verbal conflict between King and Archbishop and the Pope. When finally the exasperated King expressed his frustration, some of his courtiers interpreted this as a wish that Beckett be killed. Four knights took it upon themselves to go to Canterbury and confront the archbishop, who was about to start the service of vespers in the Cathedral. Beckett refused to listen to them and, incensed with rage, they grabbed their weapons and brutally slew him in front of the congregation. Under the rich vestments, Beckett was wearing a hair shirt. The murder shocked Christendom; Henry and the knights were forced to do penance. Here is Chaucer's prologue to his famous *Canterbury Tales*:

> Whan that aprill with his shoures soote
> The droghte of march hath perced to the roote,
> And bathed every veyne in swich licour
> Of which vertu engendred is the flour;
> And smale foweles maken melodye,
> That slepen al the nyght with open ye
> (so priketh hem nature in hir corages);
> Thanne longen folk to goon on pilgrimages,
>
> When April with his showers sweet with fruit
> The drought of March has pierced unto the root
> And bathed each vein with liquor that has power
> To generate therein and sire the flower;
> And many little birds make melody
> That sleep all the night with open eye
> (So Nature pricks them on to ramp and rage);
> Then do folk long to go on pilgrimage,

Today I reflect on arrogance and the need for true humility.

December 30th

On this day in 1865 the English writer and poet Rudyard Kipling was born. The name Kipling is almost synonymous with the British Empire and many of his finest stories such as *Kim* and *The Jungle Book* were written about India. Kipling was born in Bombay and spent many years in India. He travelled a lot but settled in Sussex with his family and died at the age of 70. Although famous for his barrack room ballads, he was never a regular soldier. He won the Nobel Prize for literature in 1907. His poem, Mandalay, is a fine example of what he does so well – it combines the mystery of the Orient with the earthy practicality of the British soldier who, at the height of the empire, might find himself on duty almost anywhere in the world.

> I am sick o' wastin' leather on these gritty pavin'-stones,
> An' the blasted English drizzle wakes the fever in my bones;
> Tho' I walks with fifty 'ousemaids outer Chelsea to the Strand,
> An' they talks a lot o' lovin', but wot do they understand?
> Beefy face an' grubby 'and –
> Law! wot do they understand?
> I've a neater, sweeter maiden in a cleaner, greener land!
> On the road to Mandalay
> Ship me somewheres east of Suez, where the best is like the worst,
> Where there aren't no Ten Commandments an' a man can raise a
>   thirst;
> For the temple-bells are callin', an' it's there that I would be
> By the old Moulmein Pagoda, looking lazy at the sea;
> On the road to Mandalay,
> Where the old Flotilla lay,
> With our sick beneath the awnings when we went to Mandalay!
> O the road to Mandalay,
> Where the flyin'-fishes play,
> An' the dawn comes up like thunder outer China 'crost the Bay!

Today I will try to understand and respect people of all races and origins.

December 31st

Today is known in the Northern regions of Britain as Hogmanay. The origins of the word and its surrounding customs are uncertain. In Scotland, Hogmanay has been the more traditional celebration since the Protestant Reformation, probably because Christmas was seen as too 'Papist'. The custom of 'first footing' and the giving of symbolic gifts such as coal, shortbread and whisky are intended to bring luck. The old English Twelve Days of Christmas, sometimes called the "Daft Days" in Scotland, are not greatly observed north of the Border. Nowadays Hogmanay is often seen as the excuse for a huge and lengthy party, with Edinburgh leading the way. This part of *The Song of Hogmanay* comes from Carmina Gadelica, the collection of Gaelic hymns and incantations made by Alexander Carmichael in the 19th century:

> *Tonight is the last night of the year,*
> *Be generous to me in the dwelling,*
> *As I come to sing my Hogmanay song,*
> *Give to me timely heed.*
> *Some at flattery, some at lies*
> *Some at words unwonted,*
> *Others devouring the gizzards*
> *Of the wheezy grey fowls;*
> *Some of them fixing their back-teeth*
> *In the black joints of the cattle,*
> *And some of them hunkering down*
> *In a corner on a heap of potatoes.*
> *I pray for you sweethearting and peace,*
> *Until a year from this time, o friends,*
> *And since my feet are bare,*
> *Open to me the fastening of the door!*

Today I reflect on the old year and look forward with hope to the next.

ABOUT THE AUTHOR

'What a Piece of Work is a Man'
Hamlet

Christopher Burn trained as an accountant and has lived in London, Paris and Malta. Over a twenty year period he successfully created an economic and cultural wilderness out of a secure and pleasant lifestyle, using only a bottle of Scotch. In 1988 he helped start Castle Craig Hospital, probably the UK's largest addiction clinic, where he remains involved to this day. At various times he has been a banker, tax adviser, taxi driver, hotelier and psychotherapist.

When the going was tough, he found solace and hope in poetry; this has been a lifelong obsession. It gave him the inspiration to start anew. Writing *Poetry Changes Lives* is his response.

Christopher is married with three children and five grandchildren. He spends his time between London and the Scottish borders.